Special Diets for Special People:

Understanding and Implementing a
Gluten-Free and Casein-Free Diet to Aid in
the Treatment of Autism and Related
Developmental Disorders

by Lisa S. Lewis, Ph.D.

Future Horizons Inc., Arlington, TX

Special Diets for Special People

All marketing and publishing rights guaranteed to and
reserved by

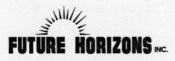

FUTURE HORIZONS INC.

721 W. Abram Street
Arlington, TX 76013

800-489-0727:

817-277-0727 817-277-2270 Fax

Website: www.FHautism.com
E-mail: info@FHautism.com

ISBN 10: 1-932565-29-9

ISBN 13: 978-1-932565-29-4

Acknowledgments

This book has evolved over a period of three years. It is extremely gratifying to see it finally completed, but I could not have done so without much help and support.

I am very grateful to the many generous cooks who graciously shared recipes. They are all credited in the preface to their own recipes, but some also helped with recipe testing, proofreading and editing chores. I thank especially Karyn Seroussi, Harriet Barnett, Barbara Crooker and Jean Jasinski for their editing and/or cooking skills. Beth Hillson of the Gluten -Free Pantry has been very helpful, and extremely generous with both information and recipes.

It is extremely fortuitous that members of my family, who cannot refuse their help, are also excellent writers and editors. Various sections of this book were read by Shelley Lewis, Stephen Lewis, Edith Rock, Bert Lewis and Serge Goldstein. All had valuable comments and criticisms which much improved the quality and clarity of my writing. My mother, Bert Lewis, took on the especially tedious task of proofreading recipes, as did my friend Jean Jasinski. I also thank members of the U.S. Rice Foundation (also known as The Rice Council) for allowing me to adapt and share their published recipes.

I am especially grateful to my guys, Serge, Sam and Jake Goldstein. They have been willing guinea pigs for many of the recipes that **didn't** make it into this book, as well as the ones that did. Sam especially enjoys the results (most) of my trials, but then, he is the least fussy of the three when it comes to food! As so often happens, having an autistic child has both broadened and narrowed our lives. Most of our pre-autism friends are gone, living "normal" lives which no longer involve us. They have been replaced with many others who know where we are coming from, like us, and worry about where we will go from here. I am so lucky to have met so many interesting and warm people. I thank them all, for sharing their own insights and feelings.

I am grateful to all the parents who have, over the last three years, called me, written to me and sent me email. I hope that this book provides some practical assistance for them, and for those who are just learning that they too, have an autistic child. I also owe a debt of gratitude to Paul Shattock, Maureen McDonnell, Dr. Bernard Rimland, Dr. Jaak Panksepp and Dr. Sid Baker, for information shared over the last several years.

Dietary and other interventions can only ameliorate autistic symptoms. We are all still waiting, not so patiently, for someone to find the cause(s) and cure for the mysterious and disabling condition. For the scientists who are working to achieve these goals I reserve my greatest respect and sincerest wishes for good luck and success in the very near future.

Lisa Lewis

Table of Contents

Foreword

I am pleased to be invited to write a foreword to this book on dietary intervention that will benefit many autistic children.

The topics have been of strong interest to me since the mid-1960s, when I began to hear from parents whose autistic children were exquisitely sensitive to certain foods. I believe the first parent from whom I heard about wheat sensitivity was Chris Griffith, who started the Georgia Chapter of the Autism Society of America, in 1966. Her severely autistic son, Joseph, showed remarkable improvement on a totally wheat-free diet. When he seized and ate the corner of a soda cracker accidentally dropped by his brother, Chris told me Joseph went out of control for four days. There followed many similar stories, from other parents. An Ohio mother reported four or five days of chaos following her son's consuming a morsel of wedding cake. ("This little bit won't hurt him.") I heard about the havoc wrought by the residue of a hamburger bun, not quite completely scraped off the meat patty by a harried mother, who had whizzed through a drive-through fast food place with her autistic son.

Then there is cow's milk—great for little cows—not so great for many autistic kids. Somewhere in my files are the letters from an Air Force family whose autistic daughter showed great improvement when the family was transferred to northern Canada, in the mid 1960s, when the father was assigned to work on the DEW system. (Note to you youngsters: DEW stands for Deployed Early Warning—a radar network designed to alert the U.S. to ballistic missiles launched across the Arctic by cold war Russia.)

On the family's return to the Midwest, when the father's DEW duty was over, the daughter's severe autism returned.

Strange! The answer: the autistic girl could tolerate reindeer milk, the only kind available, but not cow's milk!

The best-known case of autism caused by cow's milk intolerance is that of Tony, whose mother Mary Callahan told her story in her excellent book *Fighting for Tony*. Tony was clearly a case of severe autism, as the book itself and several diagnosticians attest.

Tony's pediatrician suggested a trial elimination of cow's milk to see if that might control Tony's asthma. Both his asthma and the autism disappeared when the cow's milk was taken out of his diet! On accidentally drinking cow's milk, both the asthma and autism recurred. (*Fighting for Tony* is currently out of print; however, we are working toward getting it reprinted. If you are interested, write the Autism Research Institute to see if it has become available.)

These adverse reactions to wheat and milk are commonly said to be due to allergies. However, as Dr. Lewis explains later in this book, there are technical definitions of allergic reactions, preferred by most allergists, which would exclude behavioral reactions to foods. Rather than rile these allergists, I usually refer to "food intolerance" rather than food allergies.

The only mistake I ever made (that I'm willing to own up to) was in a talk I gave on food intolerance as a cause of autism at the annual meeting of the Autism Society of America (then called NSAC—National Society for Autistic Children) in 1972. I said, to my everlasting embarrassment:

While I recognize that most physicians today are skeptical about such allergies of the nervous system, and that many have never even heard the term, I will predict that in ten to fifteen years the average physician will think of such allergies as an immediate possibility when he sees an autistic-type child, one with learning disabilities or hyperkinesis, or for that matter, an adult with migraine.

Yes, I really did say that, many years ago. Now, as I write these words, a quarter of a century has rolled by and the vast majority of physicians are still oblivious to the role food intolerance plays in causing "mental" and behavioral problems. A quick count shows over 30 books on my shelves devoted in whole or part to food intolerance causing every imaginable disorder of brain function-depression, migraine, schizophrenia, dyslexia, hyperactivity, and autism among them. At last count there were 42 journal articles solely on the link between food intolerance and autism.

Old ideas die hard and a plenitude of evidence doesn't seem to change that very much.

What will change, and is changing, the mind of the medical establishment is activist efforts by intelligent, well-informed and highly motivated parents like Mary Callahan, Lisa Lewis and many others. Enlightenment is percolating upward from the parents to the doctors, rather than trickling downward from the doctors, as the conventional model assumes.

Medical research and indifference notwithstanding, progress is being made and increasing numbers of open-minded physicians are beginning to recognize the value of looking at food intolerance as being at the root of many intractable problems, autism being only one of them. But you Moms will have to continue to lead the way.

This book is a giant step in the right direction.

Bernard Rimland, Ph.D.
Autism Research Institute

Introduction

In 1991, when he was three and a half years old, my son Samuel received a diagnosis of PDD-NOS (Pervasive Developmental Disorder—Not otherwise specified.) Although it was hard to feel lucky about *anything* that year, my husband and I quickly realized that our central New Jersey location was one of the best places in the country for facing this particular challenge. There were excellent schools and therapists available. A state group called COSAC (Community Outreach and Support for the Autistic Community) was only a few miles from our home, and through them we received invaluable information and support.

Probably because of our access to these resources, we realized sooner than most that PDD-NOS is a nonsensical label, usually used in reference to autistic children who are relatively high-functioning. Other (equally confusing) terms sometimes used are *atypical autism, mild autism* and *autistic-like*. I have even heard parents call their children "a little autistic." The term PDD-NOS has come to be most commonly used by doctors who cannot bring themselves to use the word autism when speaking to vulnerable parents[1]

Like other parents, we immediately began to have tests run and to search out new therapies. AIT (Auditory Integration Therapy) was just coming into vogue and we learned all we could about it, as well as older therapies (e.g. behavior modification, megavitamin therapy and various medications). We made contact with other parents in the area who had "been around" and while they were helpful, they were also very discouraging about progress.

At the age of five, Sam's behavior took a sudden turn for the worse, and I began grasping at straws. He was already in an excellent special school, but school personnel were grasp stumped. I tried several things, but the one thing that seemed to make a difference was removing all wheat from his diet. He had always been a good eater, but showed a real preference for anything made of flour. Since I had read that allergic children often crave the foods they should not have, I chose to eliminate wheat.[2]

We saw such improvement in Sam's behavior and demeanor, that we took him to an allergist to see what other foods might be causing him problems. To our amazement he was not allergic to any foods, including wheat! He did test positive for various pollens and molds, but showed no reaction to any food. Because this result was so puzzling, I began to research diet in the current autism literature. There wasn't much, but papers by Karl Reichelt and Paul Shattock argued that **gluten**—a protein found in wheat and other grains—was probably a significant factor.

Prior to finding these papers, I had been using oat and rye flours, and both these grains contain gluten (though in much smaller amounts than in wheat). As of November 1993, I removed **all gluten** from Sam's diet. **Although he was (and still is) a child with autism, the improvement we saw was rapid and striking.** This improvement was noticeable to everyone who knew Sam—teachers, therapists and family members. Other parents began to ask me questions about the diet he was on, how they could do the same, where to shop, how to cook, etc.

A woman I knew who had an autistic child just Sam's age asked me if I could give her some detailed instructions on how to implement this diet. Her son was having a pretty rough time, and she was desperate for any help. As a favor to her, I wrote detailed instructions on what her child should eat, where she should shop and how she should cook. I had intended to write two or three pages, but as I began writing I kept thinking of things to tell her. The paper soon grew to fifteen pages.

I had put a lot of thought and work into the paper, and decided it could be of use to many people if I did not include information pertinent only in central New Jersey. I began to rewrite the document generalizing its content and expanding upon many points. When I was done, I mentioned it on an Internet mailing list for people (mostly parents) interested in autism.[3] I had written about Sam's diet on the list before, and my postings had been largely ignored. I was thus surprised to find that requests for the document began flooding in. I did not charge for the paper, and ended up spending quite a bit of time and money to copy and mail it out. I also began getting email and phone calls from people who had heard about the paper and wanted a copy, or who had read it and wanted more information.

Eventually I rewrote the paper and put it up on a World Wide Web home page (see Appendix IV). To my surprise, the page was a big success, being seen by hundreds of people each week. The number of phone calls, letters and email I received increased, and these contacts began to come from as far away as Singapore and Malaysia! Everyone wanted more information on how to do the diet. I answered as many people as I could and within a year I had spoken with dozens of people who were in a position to make contributions to the field of autism research. I am very grateful to have heard from these people and exchange information with them; I am proud to call many of them my friends.

I have never claimed that this diet will cure autism. However, there is no doubt that the diet has had a significant, extremely beneficial effect on Sam. In the last two years I have heard from several parents of very young (less than three years old) children who have been declassified as autistic following the very early introduction of the same dietary intervention described in this book. While I am thrilled to hear of these cases, I of course regret that I didn't have this information available to me in 1991.

Because the cluster of symptoms which leads to a diagnosis of autism may have several distinct etiologies, it is unlikely that every autistic person will benefit from this diet, or any other single intervention. I believe strongly, however, that the approach *should be tried*. Current research is lending further support to the theories behind the intervention. As more parents undertake the diet there will be more data to support or refute the diet's efficacy. Since scientists and doctors put little stock in anecdotal reports, as is appropriate, it is hoped parents who try this intervention will take objective pro- and post-diet data (see Chapter 3).

In the last few years I have heard from hundreds of parents who want information about this diet...parents who want to try it, but do not know where to begin. As I started outlining information for this book, I was determined to write the book that I needed, but did not have, when I first tried a dietary approach. I have tried to clarify the underlying theories, to make them easier to understand and provide the information you need to get started. I hope I have anticipated all your questions.

I have also heard from many doctors who would like to see their patients try the diet, but cannot answer questions on the practical aspects of cooking for children on a gluten-free/casein-free (GF/CF) diet. I hope these professionals will feel that *Special Diets for Special People* is a book they can recommend to their patients.

> Final notes: Remember that no treatment will help every child. This diet is very nutritious but check with your doctor before making dramatic changes in your child's diet. Be sure to outline exactly what your child will and will not eat, so that appropriate supplements can be suggested as needed.

> Nothing presented in this book is offered as medical advice.

> I would love to hear how your child is doing. And good luck to you!

> Lisa S. Lewis, Bennington, New Jersey

Chapter 1
Sam's Story

My son Sam was born on a stormy night in June 1988. When we started for the hospital, my contractions were coming at three-minute intervals, but they had nearly stopped by the time I was finally situated in a labor room. My doctor was ready to send me home, but I simply could not bear the thought of going there, *still pregnant*. Instead, we discussed the option of breaking my water and the risk that labor would have to be induced if my contractions did not start up again within a few hours. I felt very strongly that I did not want a drug-induced labor, but I was every bit as certain that the baby and I were both ready. We decided to go for it.

As if by magic contractions began again, this time in earnest, only a few minutes after my water was broken. Three hours later, Sam made his way into our world, weighing 6 lbs.14 oz. and measuring 20 1/4 inches long.

Through nine months of pregnancy, my husband Serge had insisted that *he* was not going to be the type of father whose own life ended when his child was born. After all, he reasoned, we still had our own lives and interests. While he would love and care for the child, being a father was not going to change the fact that he had many other things he wanted to do. I never argued with Serge about this, and I never worried about his attitude. For on that early morning of June 2, 1988, Serge melted as he held his son for the first time, exactly as I had known he would. After a few moments, he looked up at me and said, "*anything* he wants." We both laughed at his sudden change of heart, but in 1988, we had no idea how little Sam would want, or how much he would need.

While my pregnancy was uneventful, our joy had been marred by the concurrent illness of Serge's father. Ten days after Sam, was born, his grandpa died. A true patriarch, Leo Goldstein s death left a great emptiness in his family. For our little family, however, sadness was lessened by Sam's presence. He was a darling baby who was very sweet and was usually smiling.

For the first year of his life Sam blossomed; a sweet, blue-eyed little munchkin who loved to cuddle, 'read' books, sing and play with us and the other children at his daycare. He reached all his early developmental milestones right on schedule, and we felt we were the luckiest people in the world.

Not everything was perfect, of course. The winter of 1988-89, Sam's first, began a series of upper respiratory infections that were invariably followed by *otitis media*—infections of the middle ear. Sam was six months old when this pattern emerged, and so began his many courses of the broad spectrum antibiotic amoxycillin. We were discouraged by this course of events, but not particularly worried. Everyone we knew, especially those who had sons rather than daughters, went through the same thing each winter. We felt lucky that at least no one had suggested surgery to implant ear tubes!

Now I look back at this period in horror, fervently wishing that I had not assumed that every cold must bring with it an ear infection. Because of this assumption, I dutifully took Sam to the pediatrician just to check, four days into every cold. And every time, he was given amoxycillin.

With spring, came a return to good health. As summer approached, Sam continued to grow into a big and increasingly attractive little boy. I grew accustomed to being stopped in stores and on the street to accept the compliments of strangers. On May 2nd, when he was exactly 11 months old, Sam began to walk. By the time his birthday rolled around he was an accomplished toddler, walking with confidence. He loved to play with us and with his babysitter's children. Sam was starting to engage in some pretend playing, picking up a school bus toy and speaking into it as though it were a phone— "Hewow Gwanma!" he would chip. Sam loved music and made up little songs whose lyrics consisted of the names of everyone close to him. We had a lovely summer—at the time not realizing that it would be the last carefree period of our lives.

As another winter was upon us, Sam descended into the same pattern of illness we had seen before. But this time it was even worse, as the infections became more severe, and moved into his lungs. When he was 18 months old Sam had a severe asthma attack, and was hospitalized for five days. In retrospect, I believe that his development was normal until shortly before that hospitalization. One of my clearest memories of this time is returning to the hospital after a short break. I had been there for four straight days, but on this night I had an important appointment so Serge took over. When I returned two hours later, Sam had finally been disconnected from his IV. He looked up at me and smiled brightly, and I realized I had not seen his cherubic face light up in several days. I remember sitting with Sam next to me, turning the pages of a Helen Oxenbury board book. For the first time ever, he named every object in the book, pointing at the same time. He had never before named *everything* in this book, and never had he said the words so clearly. He was still not completely well, but we were able to take him home the next day. My mother flew in from Nebraska to help out so that I could return to my Princeton University job.[1]

Back at home, something began to change, although we did not realize it then. There were odd little things—returning home from work my mother told me that Sam had displayed a peculiar behavior. He had walked in circles of ever-decreasing size as he listened to a favorite music cassette. It took some time but she had finally figured out what he was doing—he was following the pattern of our living room rug, and he was walking on his toes.

It was also around this time that the way Sam played began to change. Instead of stacking the rings of graduated sizes, he would spin them and laugh delightedly at their action. He lost interest in his beloved books and concentrated instead on objects that provided musical or other auditory feedback. He became obsessed with music, demanding that it be on during most of his waking hours. While he could carry a tune perfectly, he listened only to the melodies without seeming to understand that the words had any meaning. His baby-sitter still rocked him before naps, but reported that the best way to lull Sam to sleep was to put him on his back and let him watch the ceiling fan over the crib.

We weren't worried yet, focusing our concerns on the asthma and his nearly constant state of infection. But as the months passed and he approached two, questions began nagging at us. He started biting at daycare, and he seemed not to be gaining in the area of language. Some things that he had said at one time, such as "OK" for an affirmative, completely disappeared. On the other hand, as summer approached, Sam seemed better. His asthma was under control and he seemed happier and less agitated. By fall we went ahead with our plan to start him at the university affiliated daycare program.

The University N.O.W. Day Nursery is an excellent preschool with a waiting list so long that I'd enrolled Sam when I was only four months pregnant! When Sam started this program at the age of 27 months, there were other children who spoke as little as he. It was not long, however, before they passed him by. Everyone around us, including his teachers, urged us to avoid making comparisons with other children. This was very hard advice to follow; the more time we spent around this group of two-year-olds, the clearer it became that Sam was falling farther and farther behind. I recall the jolt of fear I felt during a class Christmas party when I realized that a Chinese toddler, who began the year without a single word of English, had already outpaced Sam's speech. At that same party, I first realized that Sam did not look into my eyes the way the other children did when I spoke with them. **He used to look deeply into my eyes**—when did it fade and why had I not noticed?

Most parents interested in a book such as this can relate to the denial of early development gone awry. But when I review these years as objectively as I can, I do understand why we were so reluctant to believe something was really wrong, and I can now forgive myself for missing the signs.[2] Sam was always very connected to us emotionally, and he seemed very bright from an early age. He began talking at an appropriate age, and while we acknowledged how slowly his language was progressing, we did not recognize how odd his speech was. Serge was the first to realize that Sam seemed to learn whole phrases as though they were single words. It was another two years before I understood the significance of this type of speech, when a speech therapist introduced me to the work of Dr. Barry Prizant on the subject of the "gestalt style of language processing" in autistic children.

It was a long time before I could acknowledge any of this. When I finally did I noticed something else—while Sam did speak in short sentences, he never used one that he had not already heard someone else say. Much of the time his words seemed merely to be echoing ours. Rather than responding to our words, he just repeated them much of the time. He also had a strange way of referring to himself and others—he called himself "Sam" or "you" and called other people "I." When I would say to Sam, "Do you want a Cookie?" he thought that "you" was simply another way of saying "Sam" which he could also use. He would respond, happily, "You want a cookie!" or sometimes just "want a cookie." Because I would refer to myself as "I," he seemed to think that "I" was another name for "Mommy" that he could use too. All young children go through a period of pronoun confusion, but it generally passes within a few weeks, when, amazingly, they understand the concept of shifting reference. With Sam, it did not pass, and later we learned that pronoun reversal is very common for autistic children, as is the echolalic speech we had also noticed.

Around this time, Sam began to have serious tantrums at home. His behavior was dismissed as early onset 'terrible twos' and we were labeled neurotic by friends and especially by family members (who may have been experiencing their own period of denial) when we expressed concern. Over the course of several months, however, no one could deny that Sam had problems, or dismiss them as immaturity. By the time Sam was 2 1/2, his daycare teachers expressed concern about his hearing. I knew he had excellent hearing, but believed them when they said he did not always respond to them when they called him. I had noticed the same thing at home-it sometimes seemed as if he were ignoring me. Other parents joked about 'impaired listening' as opposed to hearing impairments, but we knew there was something more going on.[3] Why was he tuning out? Sam also began to bite again—a transgression that was taken very seriously by the school.

For a nominal fee, parents could have their child screened for problems at our day nursery; of course we asked for an evaluation by the speech and language pathologist. But we were totally unprepared for the result. I wish I could remember the name of the woman who did the screening—for I owe her a great deal. She was kind, but did not mince words when she told me that Sam was severely language disordered, and probably had other developmental problems too.

She discussed specific problems we had not even noticed. She added that when she observed the whole class, Sam was the only child who drifted away from the group. He paid no attention to activities that engaged and amused the other children. According to Sam's teachers, this was not unusual behavior for him. The speech therapist suggested that I make an immediate call to Project Child (the county agency responsible for early intervention) for a full evaluation and initiation of services. I was so shocked that I stopped listening and was in fact, extremely rude.

A few days later I called her, both to apologize for my rudeness and to ask for her help. She had accomplished what no one else had been able to do—she had finally pierced through the wall of denial I had built around both Sam and me.

The therapist told me whom to call and what to ask. She drew no conclusions, although she must have had some strong opinions, judging by the forcefulness she used in getting through to me.

And so began the frustrating series of evaluations so familiar to every family with a special needs child. Our pediatrician, when asked if he thought Sam was autistic, just said "I don't know." Speech, behavioral and occupational therapists at Project Child were unwilling to assign a label to Sam, although later I realized that many thought he was autistic. All were unwilling to be the ones to tell us that they thought his problems were very serious.

As soon as a place could be found for him in the early intervention program, we began bringing him to Project Child twice a week for a few hours of therapy. Ultimately we were told that he had sensory integration difficulties, with some autistic traits. As he approached three, he was evaluated for inclusion in the county's special needs preschool. As part of that evaluation we were told that he was "definitely not autistic" based on his general responsiveness and his rapport with us and the examiners. We chose to believe this, both because we wanted to and because the (out-of-date) books I had read on the subject described children very different from our son.[4]

With summer approaching we chose to remove Sam from daycare—before we were asked to—for Serge and I were both certain this was inevitable. It was clear to all that he was not benefiting from the program, and he was a disruptive influence. Because he would be going to the county preschool the following September, it seemed reasonable to remove him from the program at that time. We hired a sitter for the summer, and

I planned to work with Sam intensively during that period (still assuming that he *could* catch up, if only we worked hard enough). We began private speech therapy and in September Sam began attending a multiply-handicapped half-day preschool.

While these classes helped Sam somewhat, his language continued to lag and he started exhibiting other troubling behaviors. He began complex stereotypies (sometimes called self-stimulatory behaviors), developed a complete insensitivity to pain, and began using peripheral vision rather than looking at objects from the center of his visual field. At a parent-teacher meeting in November, we were told that Sam "functioned at a higher cognitive level" than the other children in the class, but "demonstrated far more difficult behavior."

In general, Sam was deteriorating, falling farther behind and showing increasing numbers of abnormal behaviors. Serge was seriously worried about his adored firstborn son, sure that we did not really have the whole story. I was eight months pregnant with our second child and unable to accept or cope with what I already knew. Shortly after the birth of Sam's brother Jacob, (Sam was three and a half), Serge spent a day in the Princeton University psychology library studying the DSM-IIIR.[5] As he read through the section on autism, Serge realized he was reading a chillingly accurate description of his first born son. Despite the protestation of county professionals and our own wishes, Sam clearly belonged somewhere on the autism spectrum.

Serge came home that night, sure that I would argue with him when he told me what he had found. I did not, for I knew it was true. In a way we were both relieved to finally have a name for Sam's problems. With that name came a vindication of all the fears that had been so readily dismissed by our friends and families. More importantly, we felt that since we knew what was wrong, we would be able to find ways to 'fix' him. It wasn't long before we joined support groups and signed up for parent training. I have never forgotten the words of one father who spoke of his feelings at one of these support meetings. Of doctors he said: "First they bludgeon you with this diagnosis, and *then* they tell you there's nothing they can do about it."

Realizing that we needed a neurologist's written diagnosis to gain the services to which Sam was entitled, we went to the neurology department of the New Jersey University of Medicine and Dentistry. We answered the obligatory "What seems to be the problem?" with the words "We think he is autistic." The doctor concurred, after asking a few questions and observing Sam, and we received our 'official' diagnosis, all the while still hoping we would be told we were wrong. We had already known what was wrong with Sam; we already believed it was the right diagnosis. And yet... it *did* feel as if we had been bludgeoned with those awful words, despite the kindness of the doctor who delivered them.

At this point we felt certain that Sam's current educational placement was completely inadequate. We sought an independent educational evaluation at the Eden Institute in Princeton, New Jersey. A placement more specific to autism was recommended, and Sam was accepted at the Douglass Developmental Disabilities Center at Rutgers University for the fall. We began speech and occupational therapy at the Eden Institute's (then new) infant and toddler program. Meanwhile, we had a summer to kill, and the summer was indeed a killer.

Sam's behavior became impossible. He was extremely aggressive, and very controlling, throwing terrible fits if we did not take the car he wanted us to take, or sit where he wanted us to sit. Eden provided some desperately needed behavior therapists to work with Sam (and us) in our home. They made us realize that Sam, through his behavior, was running our home and our lives. I have no idea how we would have managed without their help.

I read everything I could find on the subject of autism. I borrowed Mary Callahan's book, *Fighting for Tony*, from Eden's small lending library. This book gave me hope—after all, she had cured her son, merely by realizing that he had a "brain allergy" to milk! I immediately removed dairy from Sam's diet, hoping that he too would be cured. His aggression decreased a little, but it remained a significant problem. Tantrums did not decrease, nor did we see other improvements. Clearly, Mary Callahan's miracle was not to be ours.

In the fall, at age four, Sam started school at Douglass. In addition to working on cognitive development and social skills, behavior modification techniques were used to eliminate his aggressive and difficult behaviors. These behavioral strategies each helped for a time, but nothing really helped for long. Douglass staff continued to search for a way to help Sam control these behaviors, as well as the stereotypies. Sam did improve a great deal in all areas during his first year at Douglass, and he remained there for four years.

Shortly after Sam's fifth birthday, his aggression suddenly increased. I had no idea what had caused it and really no clue as to what to do about it. For lack of anything else to try, and because I had recently seen Dr. Doris Rapp[6] on an afternoon talk show, I decided to experiment again with Sam's diet. I chose to remove wheat because I had learned it was one of the most common food allergens, and we had already eliminated dairy with little effect. I did not tell Sam's teachers, so they would be 'blind' to this test.

Within days of removing wheat from his diet, Sam's aggressions dropped dramatically, and I began receiving wonderful reports from school. One morning a few weeks later, I mindlessly gave Sam wheat toast for breakfast. By the time I realized what I had done, it was too late—I sent him to school and waited for the report.

When I went to get Sam off the bus, his driver told me "I heard he had a pretty rough day."[7] The report was dreadful. Within an hour of arriving at school Sam had been totally out of control. I immediately called his teacher and explained about the dietary change and the unintentional 'challenge.' From that point on we were very careful about his diet, and the school worked hard to help Sam comply.

Sam was certainly not cured—he still had tantrums and some aggressions. However, the incidence and severity dramatically decreased. We began to see other improvements as well. He was able to talk about his aggression for the first time, and he was able to learn that he could ask for a break to engage in self-stimulatory behavior if he was feeling especially tense.[8] Perhaps the most surprising change which followed soon after we removed wheat from his diet, was that his perpetually reversed pronouns suddenly straightened out!

I would never claim that Sam's gluten-free diet is the only thing that has helped him. He spent four years at Douglass, where excellent teachers and speech therapists worked with him for 11 months of the year. He also had private speech therapy for four years and private sensory integration therapy for three years. Sam wore yoke prism glasses for two years (prescribed by Dr. Mel Kaplan in Tarrytown, NY). These glasses corrected his tendency to view everything peripherally. We also worked with Sam at home, using the techniques of applied behavior analysis to continue his teaching on weekends and during school holidays.

When he was 5 1/2 tests showed that Sam had high levels of *candida* yeast. He was placed on a strict anti-yeast diet with high doses of the anti-fungal drug Nystatin, and remained on this diet for nearly nine months. We discontinued the diet because it did not seem to produce any significant benefit.

Sam continues to have difficulty with visual processing, and reading remains a real challenge for him. It is a challenge he is meeting however, and I am encouraged that Sam will read fluently in the not too distant future. His language is excellent, and he shows that he is able to generalize ideas and skills quite well. The school provides two sessions of speech, and one of Occupational Therapy each week. Noting that Sam needed and benefited from input to his vestibular system, his OT obtained a weighted vest for him. He wears it for much of each day, and teachers report it calms him down a great deal.

Not everything is wonderful, of course. Sam has shown, over the last three years, a troubling seasonal cycle. As late fall approaches, life seems to become increasingly difficult. By mid-winter we are deep into a funk which includes an increase in the number of tantrums, noncompliance and aggression. Then, as spring approaches, Sam's behavior, attitude and mood improve. It is hard to imagine this if you have not observed it, but the decline in his performance and behavior during winter is quite extreme. Each spring we grew hopeful that we could move him from the highly restrictive school he attended, only to have hopes dashed as we began the down cycle.

We have, of course, consulted many professionals and experimented with many different factors to determine what could be causing this seasonal fluctuation. I even bought the full spectrum lamp prescribed for people who have seasonal affective disorders. He loved his lamp, but it did not help him.

As Sam's fourth year at Douglass was nearing an end, we felt certain that he simply did not belong there anymore. For the majority of each school year, it was not an appropriate setting for him. But we were very concerned that Sam would be kept in this highly restrictive school, due to the behaviors that appeared each winter. This presented us with a real quandary about starting Sam on medications. We had always strived to help Sam without drugs, but the time had come to weigh the benefit of having him experience a less restrictive school environment, against our reluctance to use medication.

Ultimately, we decided that medication was the lesser of two evils, and we found one that, for the most part, turned his winters around. A small dose of the atypical neuroleptic drug Risperdal (Risperidone) could 'get him through' this portion of the year with relatively few problems. Even *with* medication Sam was, and even now, is not at his best during winter. It does, however, reduce problem behaviors to a level that we can all handle.

Initially, we planned to use this medication only during the difficult part of the year, but we have found that Sam does better and is happier when he takes it. We have found that a 'drug vacation' of at least a few weeks is necessary to maintain the effectiveness of the drug at a low dose. I wish I did not have to use medication at all, but for now, Sam does better and seems much happier when he takes it. He also takes many supplements including vitamins, minerals, amino acids and evening primrose oil.

As of this writing, Sam continues to grow and improve, and has developed into a friendly, sociable little boy. I realize that these adjectives are not readily applied to a child with autism, but they are quite accurate descriptions of him.

Last year, Sam was gradually transitioned into a district school, with a great deal of support and instruction from the staff of his former school and began attending this "regular" school full time, with a personal aide trained by the Douglass staff. Sam did his academic work in a self-contained, special education classroom with one-on-one attention from his teacher or aide. He attended morning meeting, art, music, gym, lunch, recess and other 'specials' with his second grade peers, and it is these peers whom Sam now regards as his friends.

Sam's attendance at school required many adjustments on the part of school personnel. Serge worked with the children at the start of the school year so they could understand Sam's struggles better, and these children continue to show patience and a willingness to help Sam whenever they can. In our small, very homogeneous community, these children have benefited from Sam's presence. They have learned that some people are different than they are, and must face completely different challenges in life. This is a hard lesson to learn, but perhaps the world would be a better place if we all came to this understanding at so tender an age. Of course, no one has benefited from the experience as much as Sam, who is thrilled to be there and happy to have peers who respond to him.

So...how will this story end? Will Sam become an independent adult? Will he get through school? Hold down a job? Will he have real friends who share his interests? At this point, I really don't know. What is certain is that Sam improves, steadily if slowly, every day. We will continue to do whatever is needed to ensure that Sam becomes the best that he can be. And whatever happens, we will love him for himself, and for all the struggles he has and will certainly endure in the future.

Chapter Two
About Special Diets

The idea of using a special diet to treat a child with autism is, on the surface, a rather unconventional approach to treatment. After all, autism is known as a 'pervasive" developmental disability with seemingly little to do with nutrition or food.

In fact, it is only after living or working with autistic children that one can really appreciate how pervasive autism truly is. It is a disorder that affects and disables many of the very characteristics by which we humans define ourselves. Autism affects how a person relates to other people and to the world. It impairs the ability to use sophisticated language, with roughly one third of individuals with autism never able to speak at all.[1] Autism affects a person's basic understanding of how the world operates and what accommodations we must each make to live peaceably within society. In many (perhaps most) cases, autism affects intelligence. (59)

Why would anyone think a diet could help a disorder as pervasive as autism? The answer to that question is complicated with much of the explanation still speculative.

People have used dietary interventions to treat diseases for many years but, as one might expect, this approach is rarely attempted when more conventional medical interventions are already available. Bluntly stated, dietary interventions are almost always tried for disorders that are, at the time, incurable. When no pharmaceutical or surgical treatments are available, diets may be tried out of desperation, from the perspective that "We might as well give *this* a shot." And while not all dietary interventions have been successful, many have produced significant improvement in specific symptoms.

The **"Ketogenic diet"** is a good example of a diet used to treat a medical problem that seems to bear no relation to food or nutrition. Seventy years ago, doctors at Johns Hopkins Hospital in Baltimore began using an extremely high fat, low protein and carbohydrate diet to manage seizure disorders. They were inspired by the discovery in ancient times, that 'fits' were often cured temporarily by fasting. The Ketogenic diet lost popularity many years ago but resurfaced in the 1990's when Dr. John Freeman and nutritionist Millicent Kelly wrote a book on the use and management of the diet. (20) It is again being used at medical centers around the country to control intractable epileptic seizures in patients who do not respond to conventional drug therapy and are not good candidates for surgery. Recently it has been used for children with infantile seizures.

In the Ketogenic diet, fat becomes the main energy source for the body (much like the Atkins weight loss diet). When dietary fat is used for energy, ketone bodies are produced as a byproduct of fat metabolism. It is believed that ketones inhibit seisure activity, although the precise mechanism by which this occurs is not understood. It is believed that anywhere from 50-75% of children put on this diet show considerable improvement in the control of their seizures. (21)

Despite the fact that all anti-seizure medications have the potential for serious side effects, doctors do not typically provide information about dietary intervention unless at least two of these medications have not worked. Even when medications dull the young patients into virtual insensibility, many doctors strongly discourage trying the diet if the seizures are under control. In March 1994, the news magazine show *Dateline NBC* aired a report on the Ketogenic diet, bringing the diet 'out of the closet'. When asked on-air why most doctors don't tell patients about the Ketogenic diet Dr. Donald Shields of UCLA'S pediatric neurology department stated bluntly that 'no one profits, since there are no costly drugs to dispense."

Most allopathic doctors give other reasons for resisting this treatment option. Most notably, they cite the lack of large scale, controlled clinical trials and the difficulty of following the diet. (21) Even though these reasons may be valid, many parents are now enrolling their children In hospital-based diet programs,[2] hoping to control the seizures without turning their children into drug-induced zombies.

Doctors are correct that the diet is hard to follow. It should only be tried under a doctor's care, and must be managed very carefully. Food needs to be weighed and the diet MUST be strictly adhered to. Responders generally remain seizure free after being weaned from the Ketogenic diet, typically after a period of one to three years. (21) For parents who are interested in learning more about this intervention, there are web sites and news groups on the Internet devoted to discussion of the Ketogenic diet (see Appendix IV).

Another example of a successful dietary treatment relates to **recurrent respirator papillomatosis (RRP)**, a rare disease in which tumors grow inside the larynx, vocal chords and trachea. (10) According to a 1995 study, approximately 2,350 new pediatric cases and 3,600 new adult cases were diagnosed in the U.S. during a one-year period. The Human Papilloma Virus (HPV) is present in these respiratory tumors, and the tumors are called papillomas. (61) These growths are often associated with two specific types of the virus (HPV6 and HPV11), which are also found in genital and cervical warts. Although it is not known for certain, many researchers believe that transmission of the disease may occur at the time of birth. If a mother has these warts, the baby can be exposed to the virus as it passes through the birth canal. (10)

Growing papillomas can obstruct the airway, and suffocation will likely occur if the tumors are left untreated. Because of this risk, the main focus of treatment has been the removal of the tumors by CO_2 laser surgery, under general anesthesia. Such surgery merely alleviates the problem for a time. While periods of spontaneous remission are well documented the disease does return. When the disease is active the result can be dozens of surgeries within a very short period of time. Each time surgery is performed there is, along with the risks of the anesthesia, increasing risk that the patient's ability to speak normally will be compromised. (61)

For RRP patients, there have been few advances in treatment options. Interferon has been tried, but it has many side effects and there is concern that its use can cause a rebound effect in the disease (eventually causing an increase in tumor growth). Photodynamic therapy, which for some patients lengthened the period between recurrences of tumor growth, causes an extreme sensitivity to light, however, and other worrisome side effects. Acyclovir, a medicine that has provided great benefits to sufferers of shingles and genital herpes, *seemed* to help some RRP patients; this is quite puzzling, since it affects an enzyme in the herpes virus that isn't present in the papilloma virus. A follow-up study later showed Acyclovir to be ineffective for RRP.

In 1992, however, doctors at Long Island Jewish Medical Center began testing a very interesting treatment protocol for RRP, which had no side effects at all. Oddly, the treatment did not even include medication, but was based on cabbage juice. (10)

Why cabbage juice? It is known that there are two distinct metabolic pathways for estrogen, one of which produces an estrogen metabolite that worsens the RRP tumors. Doctors now believe that there is a relationship between a compound found in Cruciferous vegetables (e.g. cabbage, broccoli, cauliflower and brussel sprouts) and estrogen metabolism. This compound, indole-3-carbonal (I3C) seems to induce estrogen metabolism via the 'good' pathway and shunt it away from the 'bad' pathway. (27)

This was at first merely a theory, but further study has shown that there is a strong linear relationship between the ratio of the two estrogen metabolic pathways and the severity of the RRP. In other words, the higher the percentage of estrogen that is metabolized by the 'bad' pathway, the more severe the disease. Doctors hoped that by increasing dietary intake of the I3C compound, RRP patients could force more estrogen metabolism to occur via the 'good' pathway. (27)

Initially, patients were told to take two cups of Cruciferous vegetables a day, but it was hard to determine how much of the significant compounds were being taken. It was also hard to eat that much cabbage! Later, it was determined that juicing the vegetables allowed for easier measurement of the necessary compounds. Since cabbage juice isn't all that palatable (especially to children) it was recommended that the cabbage juice be mixed with fruit juices. (27) Although the sample sizes are too small to make definitive statements about this therapy, more this half the respondents in a recent survey of therapies for RRP showed very significant improvement. Some patients following this protocol have been in remission for over five years. The necessary compounds can now be obtained in a supplement, so RRP patients no longer need to eat or drink large volumes of vegetables. (61)

Another disorder for which dietary interventions have been used is **Attention Deficit Hyperactivity Disorder (ADHD).** Although estimates vary, most agree that the diagnosis of ADHD is nearing epidemic proportions in American schools. (64) Some reports place the number of school age children taking stimulant medication at over two million! (2) As is true for most learning and developmental disabilities, boys with this disorder outnumber girls by a ratio of approximately 5:1. These children have various problems, including distractibility, impulsiveness and hyperactivity. The behaviors of the disorder generally become noticeable at school age, and include difficulty remaining seated and paying attention, difficulty obeying instructions, shifting from one uncompleted activity to another, difficulty playing quietly, talking excessively, interrupting, losing things, and being unaware of the consequences of their actions. (47)

The vast majority of ADHD children are placed on stimulant medication. Drugs such as Methylphenidate (Ritalin) and Pemoline (Cylert) are generally recognized as safe, but many parents believe that their children's behavior *could* be dealt with without resorting to the use of stimulants. (47) Despite potential risks and over the objections of most parents, many teachers have begun to *insist* that these boisterous children not be allowed in their classroom unless medication is used to make them quieter and more compliant.

Even when a neurological disorder is clearly causing the active and distracting behaviors, many parents would rather limit medication if at all possible. There is also evidence that these medications promote motor tics such as those seen in people with Tourette's Syndrome. (2) Many children with ADD, ADHD or autism appear to be at increased risk for developing these tics, and the benefit of stimulants should be weighed carefully against these potential problems.

For parents of ADHD children, Dr. Ben Feingold came along as a white knight in 1975, when he published *Why Your Child is Hyperactive*. (19) The late Dr. Feingold was a pediatric allergist in San Francisco who claimed that childhood hyperactivity was caused by food dyes, artificial flavorings and certain preservatives commonly used to increase the shelf life of foods. He pointed out that over 80% of the food additives in our nation's food supply[3] were artificial colors and flavors.

Feingold hypothesized a genetically mediated sensitivity to certain artificial ingredients, citing the direct correlation between the increasing use of additives and the rise in learning and behavior problems. He prescribed a diet that eliminated these items, as well as foods containing the natural chemicals known as salicylates (salicylates are found in almonds, apples, apricots, berries, cherries, cucumbers, grapes, oranges, plums, tangerines and tomatoes). (19)

Dr. Feingold believed that two distinct pathways are involved when children eat foods containing additives and dyes. He called the first of these the "toxic pathway." Molecules can cross the blood-brain barrier, which is designed to prevent large molecules from passing into the brain or spinal cord from the blood—after escaping intact from the intestine to the bloodstream. Once in the brain, these molecules can cause neurological problems by interfering with the chemical and electrical functioning of the brain. (19)

The second important biochemical pathway involved is immunological and comes into play when a food allergy exists and a reactive food is eaten. Allergic responses can reduce the levels of neurotransmitters;[4] with this reduction, behavioral changes can be expected. (19,60)

Whether or not food additives are causing behavioral problems for children diagnosed as ADD or ADHD is still controversial. C.H.A.D.D., the world's largest support and information network for children and adults with ADHD, at this time regards dietary therapy as "experimental".

Subsequent articles have supported dietary intervention. A 1994 article in *Annals of Allergy* showed that children who eliminated wheat, dairy, corn soy, citrus, eggs, chocolate, artificial colors and preservatives experienced far less hyperactivity than they had previously—when their diets returned to "normal" their behavior regressed. (5) A 1994 study published in the *Journal of Pediatrics* reported on a double-blind study of the effect of food colors and additives on behavior. (51) This study supports the dietary intervention, as do the anecdotal reports of thousands of parents. Several practitioners have also had good success treating these symptoms with homeopathic medications. Some related autism research also supports the thesis that dietary intervention is helpful for many children diagnosed with ADD and ADHD. (35,56) (Many of the recipes in Part II of this book may be easily adapted to the Feingold regimen.)

While mainstream medicine considers dietary intervention to be controversial for the ADD and ADHD population, a special diet is the *only* accepted treatment for **Celiac Disease (CD)**. (3,9) CD (also known as Celiac Sprue or Gluten Sensitive Enteropathy) is a chronic disease in which the ingestion of gluten causes a characteristic type of lesion in the small intestine. The destruction of the gut wall causes improper and incomplete nutrient absorption and children with this disease typically show serious gastrointestinal problems, fatty stools and slow growth. Since only recently have researchers determined that many patients with a gluten sensitivity serious enough to damage the gut wall show *no such symptoms in childhood*, it is likely that there are a great number of undiagnosed celiac children. In CD patients, all sources of gluten must be completely eliminated from the diet. (9)

A disorder very closely related to celiac disease, and necessitating the same dietary intervention, is a skin disease known as **dermatitis herpetiformes (DH).** Dermatitis herpetiformes is a skin manifestation of gluten sensitivity and 70-80% of DH patients have coexisting damage in the intestine. In many cases DH sufferers have no signs of intestinal difficulty, and yet at least 70% actually do suffer from CD! (3)

DH appears as a bumpy rash, usually on the arms, legs or buttocks. It is extremely itchy and may also burn. Since few pediatricians have seen DH, it is most likely called eczema or atopic dermatitis when it first presents. The cortisone creams prescribed by these doctors don't relieve itching or heal the rash. While there are medications that help, the elimination of gluten from the diet is the only way to prevent its reoccurrence. (3)

To fully understand the diet which *must* be used by individuals with celiac disease and DH, and which is advocated here for autism and other pervasive developmental disorders, it is important to know more about gluten. **What *is* Gluten?** Glutens are proteins found in the Plant Kingdom Subclass of *Monocotyledonae*, the grass family of wheat, oats, barley, rye and triticale. Derivatives of these grains include: malt, grain starches, hydrolyzed vegetable/plant proteins, textured vegetable proteins, grain vinegar, soy sauce, grain alcohol, flavorings and the binders and fillers found in vitamins and medications. (3,13,49)

Avoiding gluten, and a similar dairy protein called casein, is at the heart of the dietary intervention outlined in this book. The reasons for adopting this diet will become clear in the sections and chapters to follow; what will also become clear is how difficult it is to actually avoid this protein. The short list of grain derivatives in the above paragraph belies the fact that gluten is present everywhere in the typical American diet. To fully understand why the removal of gluten, and the structurally similar dairy protein casein, is important, we need to start with some background information about autism research.

Autism

In the early 1980's, it was noted that the behavior of animals under the influence of opioid drugs such as morphine, was very similar to that of some people with autism. (42) Dr. Jaak Panksepp proposed that autistics *might* have elevated levels of naturally occurring opioids in their Central Nervous System. (41) There are several naturally occurring opioid compounds; the best known being the beta-endorphins, which produce the so-called 'runner's high'. At about the same time, work by Swedish autism expert Christopher Gillberg showed elevated levels of "endorphin like substances" in the cerebro-spinal fluid of some autistics.(25) It is particularly interesting to note that levels are high in autistic children who are insensitive to pain and who engage in self-injurious behaviors.

Norwegian scientist Karl Reichelt found abnormal peptides in the urine of people with autism; these peptides are apparently similar to those found by Gillberg. (31,45,46) Reichelt's findings were later replicated by the Autism Research Unit at the University of Sunderland under the direction of Paul Shattock. (53-56, 67) According to Shattock, "In the urine of about 50% of people with autism there appear to be elevated levels of substances with properties similar to those expected from opioid peptides." (54)

Because the level of urinary compounds greatly exceeds what could possibly be of CNS origin, researchers presumed they resulted from the incomplete breakdown of certain foods. Proteins consist of long chains of amino acids. Normally, intestinal enzymes digest them, breaking the bonds that connect the amino acids. However, genetic mutations, caused by changes in DNA, can result in specific intestinal enzymes being unable do their work.

Enzymes are also proteins; they too consist of long chains of amino acids, which fold into specific three-dimensional shapes. Each enzyme has an active site into which fits the protein it is designed to digest. If through genetic mutation an enzyme is altered, it may fold in a new way, and the protein no longer fits into the active site. (11) "Mutations...can change the chemistry of the body by preventing or altering the way certain enzymes and chemical reactions work." (11)

When this happens, the incomplete digestive process leaves amino acids bound into short chains called **peptides**. Two commonly ingested proteins are known to break down into peptides that have opioid activity: casein and gluten. **Casein**, a protein in cow's milk, breaks down to produce a peptide called *casomorphin*, and **gluten** from wheat, rye, oats and barley breaks down to form *gliadinomorphin*. (22) If the enzymes designed to digest wheat and milk are not functioning properly, the resulting peptides could still be biologically active—that is, they could function as opioids (supporting Panksepp's observations and explaining some of the symptoms we see in autism). When this happens, most of the peptides are normally dumped harmlessly into the urine. But if some of these peptides escape the gut and enter the bloodstream, they could cross the blood-brain barrier, causing serious neurological problems. (53,54,67)

Ongoing research performed by Shattock's group in England has focused on urine sample analysis using the High Performance Liquid Chromatographic (HPLC) technique. This technique has been used, with frequent improvements, for over ten years to study the urine samples of autistic individuals. HPLC separates peptides present in the urine, and produces the results graphically, which facilitates analysis. Each of the peptides shows up as a peak on a graph; each peak represents the time when a peptide was visible in the experiment. The various peptides are known to appear within a very specific time frame, and by graphing when the peaks appear, scientists can determine which peptides are present.

Analysis of urine of autistic people has shown two main peaks which are not present (or if present, are not nearly as large) in the urine of normal controls. The first peak has been identified as beta-casomorphin (from milk). The second peak was initially suspected to represent a gluten derived peptide. However, this was very puzzling, since children who had been completely gluten-free for long periods still showed this distinctive second peak. It has only recently been identified as **trans Indolyl-Acryloyl Glycine** (tIAG.)[5] (56)

Shattock *et. al.* believe that tIAG represents the detoxified version of a parent compound, Indolyl Acrylic Acid (IAA.) IAA is detoxified by the addition of the amino acid glycine. The presence of tIAG in the system strongly suggests that IAA was also present. If correct, this finding is important, since the presence of IAA can have profound effects on the permeability of various membranes, including that of the gut. (56)

Because the compounds that comprise tIAG are not all amino acids, tIAG cannot accurately be called a peptide. However, the two main elements of the molecule are joined by a peptide bond. One element (glycine) is an amino acid. The other, indole, is not an amino acid, but is believed to be derived from another amino acid, tryptophan. Shattock's group coined the word "peptoid" when referring to tIAG, since it seems to behave as a peptide though, strictly speaking, it is not one.

One credible interpretation of Shattock's research is that tIAG's presence is a significant indicator of membrane leakiness, especially of the gut and blood brain barrier. If correct, levels of other peptides may indicate the presence of biologically active peptides in the urine and the body. It follows that if the body cannot properly digest food proteins into their constituent amino acids, the remaining peptides would be able to pass through this extremely leaky gut, enter the bloodstream and pass through the blood-brain barrier. (56)

We do not yet understand why so many autistic people are unable to break down these proteins. A deficiency in one or more enzymes required for proper metabolism would seem a likely explanation, but if true this deficiency has yet to be discovered. We know from our understanding of the disease Phenylketonurea (PKU) that the effect of such a deficiency can be very profound. If indole is indeed derived from tryptophan, there could be an enzyme deficiency involved in the metabolism of this amino acid.

If this, or a similar theory ultimately explains the presence of tIAG and its significance to the incomplete breakdown and dispersal of these peptides, perhaps safe and effective supplementation can be found to prevent damage to the gut and the resulting neurological problems. Until we know for certain what is causing these problems, we must look for other ways to counteract their effects and find strategies for reducing the impact of opioids on neurological damage.

One approach is the anti-opioid drug naltrexone. Naltrexone has shown very mixed results, however, as there are difficulties associated with its administration. (8,55) Finding the optimal dose is difficult, and it is a very bitter pill, which most children will resist taking. A second approach is the complete exclusion of casein and gluten from the diet. According to Reichelt, casein is most significant for children who display autistic traits in infancy. (personal communication) Children who develop normally until a later age (18 months-two years) probably are more sensitive to gluten, which is introduced much later than milk and early solid foods. The elimination of both gluten and casein is generally recommended, however, because the amino acid sequence of the two molecules are extremely similar. (45,46)

Many parents have had traditional allergy tests run, and most report that the results did not indicate their children were allergic to wheat or milk. (53) This is probably true. Children who are helped by a GL/CF diet are generally not allergic in the traditional sense; they are gluten or casein *intolerant*. According to Shattock, "The results are akin to poisoning rather than an extreme sensitivity such as occurs in celiac disease or sensitivity to certain food colorings." (53)

Some children initially suffer a bad reaction to the removal of their favorite foods. Often, this group of children seems nearly addicted to a specific type of food—consuming large quantities of dairy or wheat products. (45) They may do very well for a few days, then suffer a regression. According to Reichelt, this bodes well for the success of the intervention. Once this period passes, it is generally followed by a good response. (31,32,45) Younger children are more likely to benefit dramatically from this intervention, but I have heard from several adults who removed gluten and casein from their diets; most report improved concentration and lessened sensory scrambling. (personal communication)

Celiacs who have not begun following a gluten-free diet have an excessively porous intestinal wall—sometimes called a "leaky gut." A damaged gut means that nutrients cannot be properly absorbed, and sufferers are often malnourished and sickly. In addition, imperfections in the gut wall allow large molecules that should be contained by the gut wall to escape into the bloodstream. (3,9) This could be the way in which improperly digested reptiles pass into the bloodstream and then cross the blood-brain barrier. (6,14-16,25,26) If these reptiles also have opioid activity, neurological problems could result. Thus, the speculation that CD is present in some autistic children who benefit from a gluten-free diet is not inconsistent with the opioid excess theory of Reichelt and Shattock.[6]

In CD patients, there is also often a difficulty in digesting milk products, but it is believed that this is due to the lactose (sugar) in milk rather than true casein (protein) intolerance. (3,8,40) Many celiacs find that after their gut has healed, they can once again consume dairy products.

While no one claims to know the cause of all cases of autism, few claim a causal role for gluten or other protein intolerance. (50,62) However, gluten exists as a 'hidden ingredient' in many foods, medicines, and even in the envelope glue we lick. It is possible that autistic children put on a so-called gluten-free diet were inadvertently ingesting gluten in minute amounts. For people with full-blown Celiac Disease, even tiny amounts can be toxic; it is not far-fetched to imagine that in less severe forms of gluten intolerance, minute amounts could also cause harm. When full-blown CD is diagnosed, it can take more than a month on a gluten-free diet to see changes in health; again, it is not far-fetched to assume that the same is true for people with gluten intolerance that have different outward symptoms. (3) It may be that early researchers and parents who tried this intervention simply gave up too soon to see these changes.

Patients with full-blown CD often have terrible symptoms of gastrointestinal distress, fatigue, and failure to grow or gain weight. (3,8,50) Because these symptoms are not easily ignored, diagnosis can be made and the diet changed when the child is relatively young. But it is possible that far less severe forms of CD exist and are, in fact, quite common. If left undiagnosed for years, the toxic effects of ingested gluten could prove extremely damaging, perhaps even causing permanent damage to the central nervous system.

In an article cited in a recent newsletter of the American Celiac Society, Dr. Allessio Fasano wrote:

> In recent years there has been a noticeable change in the age of onset of symptoms and the clinical presentation of celiac disease. Because the typical symptoms of gastrointestinal dysfunction are frequently absent in older children, the diagnosis beyond the first two years of life is more difficult and often delayed. These cases are now regarded as having atypical or late onset forms of celiac disease.

Dr. Bernard Rimland and Meyer noted thirty years ago, that children with the highest scores on Rimland's E-2 Diagnostic Checklist for autism also showed many gastrointestinal symptoms. (48) It has also been suggested that CD is an autoimmune disorder with gluten stimulating increased synthesis of some antibodies in CD patients. (50) Ruth Sullivan noted that "though few children with celiac disease have autism, it seems a disproportionate number of autistic children have celiac. Why? Does malabsorption of the small intestine prohibit vital substances (like serotonin...) from reaching the brain? If so, why do not all 'classic cases' have celiac? Or do they?" (62)

Recent studies by Dr. Rosemary Waring, of the University of Birmingham, UK, have turned up evidence that autistic children have a marked deficiency in an enzyme group called **Phenol Sulfur transferase (PST).** (35,39,65,66) It has since been determined that children with a range of learning problems also have a deficiency in this vital enzyme group. What does this mean? To understand the significance of this finding a little background biochemistry is helpful.

The PST system is one of the body's major means of detoxification. In a recently published book, Dr. Sidney Baker describes the PST system very succinctly:

This system helps us get rid of leftover hormones, neurotransmitters and a wide variety of other toxic molecules. Some such molecules come from our own metabolism, like leftover hormones and neurotransmitters, and some come into us with our food or are made by the germs that live in our intestines. (Detoxification & Healing: The Key to Optimal Health, 1997). (1)

As stated by Dr. Baker, PST is necessary to break down hormones, some food components and toxic chemicals. If the PST system is dysfunctional, the body cannot detoxify itself—that is, it will be unable to render these substances harmless. Harmful substances which should be metabolized would then build up to abnormal levels—these substances include serotonin, dopamine and noradrenaline, all of which are important neurotransmitters. In addition, many other metabolic processes can be disturbed by phenolic compounds and may cause physical problems that were not previously thought to be associated with autism—excessive thirst, night sweating, facial flushing, reddened ears. In fact, many children who test positive for PST deficiency show these types of symptoms in addition to autism. (1)

We are constantly subjected to toxic substances, some from our own metabolism, and others introduced from the outside (e.g. environmental pollutants). In detoxification, toxins are changed into harmless substances that can be excreted from the body. The process of 'disarming' these toxins often involves transforming the toxin into another substance altogether. Often this information is accomplished by adding a molecule to a toxic one, making the original one larger but benign. The detoxification process is called **conjugation**. (1,35,60)

Sulfate conjugation is one such process, required for the transformation of many chemicals in our bodies, including many drugs, phenolic compounds and neurotransmitters. For sulfate conjugation to occur, the chemical process must be started, or catalyzed, by a specific enzyme. There are many enzymes in our bodies that serve this critical function, with PST the principal enzyme group responsible for catalyzing the sulfate conjugation of neurotransmitters. A failure in this system can occur if there is a deficiency of the sulfur transferals enzyme, but it will also occur if there are not enough sulfate ions needed to accomplish the process. Waring's data suggest that it is an insufficient number of sulfate ions which causes problems for autistics. (60,65)

A large proportion of neurotransmitters are sulfate conjugated; the enzymes needed to catalyze the process are therefore of critical importance. PST is also vital to the sulfate conjugation of phenolic compounds. This is an important point, for we are literally surrounded by phenols. (24) They are nearly everywhere in the foods we eat and juices we drink. They are present in detergents and other household chemicals, even in freshly cut grass! If the PST system is deficient, it will become overburdened; the detoxification of neurotransmitters and other toxins will not be accomplished. (39,60,65,66)

The children most likely to show PST deficiency (based on Waring's small sample size) showed normal development for the first 18 months to two years of life, and also showed family histories of asthma, skin problems and migraine. (39) Typically these children also showed a sensitivity to foods and food additives which contain many phenols of many types e.g. wheat, milk, artificial pigments, artificial colors and salicylates. (35)

Unfortunately, there is no standardized, recommended treatment for PST deficiency. Two approaches may be taken— *increase* the body's ability to detoxify itself or *decrease* the toxic load to which it is subjected. Neither approach is particularly easy or 100% effective. To quote Developmental Delay Registry Founder and Nutritionist Kelly Dorfman, "Unfortunately, no amount of intervention...can totally unburden PST...enzymes...That is why it is critically important to improve the efficiency of the faulty enzyme system while attempting to lessen the load." (17) One way to 'lessen the load' is to eliminate food components that require the precious sulfate ions for detoxification. In other words, don't 'waste' this limited resource on removing compounds from the body that can, without too much trouble, be avoided. (17)

Why bother with restricting the diet? Wouldn't it make more sense simply to **add sulfate** through supplementation? Unfortunately, sulfate ions are not absorbed from the gut. Since the amino acid cysteine is the main source of free sulfate in the body, some parents have given children very large amounts of it, but this did not appear to help. (55) Others have attempted to reduce problems by supplementing with Taurine, which has been reported as having an anti-opioid effect. (7) Another approach is to supplement with methionine, another sulfur-bearing amino acid.[7] (1,7)

It is significant that the artificial colorings, preservatives and salycilates forbidden by the Feingold diet are all highly phenolic compounds; it may turn out that the ADD and ADHD children who have responded favorably to this regimen are those with PST deficiencies. By eliminating salycilates and other highly phenolic food additives, Dr. Feingold clearly unburdened the toxic load being carried by the child's system.

After hearing a talk by Dr. Rosemary Waring on the topic of PST deficiency, Sandra O. Johnson devised *Sara's Diet*. (28) This 'white diet' eliminates all artificial and natural pigments to reduce the load on the PST system as completely as possible. Although some foods are eventually returned to the diet, the regimen is extremely restrictive. In Kelly Dorfman's words:

Some parents have used diets that remove all known phenol compounds (such as Sara's Diet) to take pressure off the PST...system. While sometimes helpful, these diets are extraordinarily difficult to implement long-term as naturally occurring phenols are in every food with color. Except in extreme cases, a diet reducing toxic load from the most concentrated sources...appears to be the best. That is, reduce juices (or limit to pear juice) and eliminate all artificial colors and flavors. (17)

As word of PST deficiency spread, many autism researchers were intrigued by the suggestion that it could cause improper metabolism of neurotransmitters. It has been known for years that autistics often have abnormal levels of serotonin, as measured in the blood. The buildup of serotonin is interesting and may prove to be very significant upon further research. Another equally interesting point is the effect a PST deficiency would have on the permeability of the intestinal lining.

The proteins lining the gut are normally sulfated, and form a protective layer over the surface of the gut wall. If sulfating is deficient, proteins can clump together, causing gaps in the gut wall, and providing a good gateway through which improperly metabolized proteins could escape into the bloodstream. Since these proteins have been shown to have opioid activity, neurological problems would most likely result.

Although most of the reports are anecdotal, there is very good evidence that a diet eliminating gluten and/or casein may indeed be extremely beneficial. In a 1996 article, Waring and Reichelt stated, "We think that the demonstrated peptides may be central to the etiology of the disease. Exorphins not only increase social isolation in animal models, but may cause CNS inhibition of maturation." (66) Put more simply, the opioid peptides in question may stunt normal central nervous system development. Another observation is equally intriguing: "...because most bioactive peptides are found in different chain lengths, but with very similar activity, different peptidase defects would cause similar but not identical symptom profiles and peptide profiles." In other words, there could be several different genetic flaws affecting different enzymes that would result in the same symptoms.

For the parents of developmentally delayed or disabled children, the medical history nearly always includes a series of ear infections and antibiotic treatment. Many parents say their children "practically lived on antibiotics" and indeed, many were even put on prophylactic (preventive) doses for periods of months or even years. But while most children fed this diet of antibiotics developed normally, the vast majority of atypical children did ingest the medications, and continued to show, as they matured, severely disordered immune systems.

According to Michael Schmidt, Lendon Smith and Keith Sehnert, doctors simply are not taught alternatives to antibiotic dosing in medical school. (52)

A basic tenet of allopathic medicine is that infections are due to organisms (bacteria, viruses or parasites). Organisms can be killed with antibiotics. Therefore, infections should be treated with antibiotics. This view has changed little in the past fifty years despite evidence that the underlying theory is fragmentary and insufficient to explain why we succumb to these organisms. (52)

Antibiotic abuse is rampant, even in situations where their usefulness is questionable. Broad-spectrum antibiotics (e.g. Amoxycillin, Keflex, Ceclor, Bactrim and Septra) are nearly always prescribed for ear infections. Many (if not most) ear infections clear up without treatment. More importantly, these drugs wipe out normal intestinal flora which can enable the population of normally occurring yeasts to expand dramatically. (12,57-58)

When treatment really is necessary, doctors sensitive to these problems prescribe drugs such as penicillin or erythromycin, rather than a broad-spectrum drug. Such (rare) doctors will also prescribe a short course of an anti-fungal agent such as Nystatin. Obtaining a prescription for an anti-fungal drug will likely be an uphill battle with most doctors. While they will readily admit that the drugs being prescribed will cause gastrointestinal upsets and vaginal yeast infections in women, they still laugh at the notion that an overgrowth of yeast in the gut after taking antibiotics might cause illness.

Many doctors claim that the overuse of antibiotics is the fault of their patients, who insist on medicine when they or their children are ill. This is probably true; doctors are not the only ones raised with this model of treatment. However, doctors who knowingly prescribe an antibiotic to treat a viral infection to satisfy a patient's demand are not behaving responsibly. It would only take a few moments to explain that currently available medicines won't help a viral infection, and to suggest some other non-pharmaceutical treatments to alleviate discomfort. If doctors continue to prescribe medications they know will not help a child's illness, it is up to parents to resist the temptation to ask for medication.

In addition to weakening the immune system's ability to recognize and fight off bacterial infection, the abuse of antibiotics has led to strains of antibiotic resistant bacteria. (52) Doctors often must look for new or stronger antibiotics to prescribe for bacterial infections, because older ones no longer work.

Dr. William Crook of Jackson, Tennessee, has long championed the notion that abuse of antibiotics has damaged children. He believes that a vicious cycle begins when an upper respiratory or ear infection is treated with antibiotics. The antibiotic throws off the balance of the intestinal flora by killing off 'good' bacteria, which provide protection against fungal and parasitic infections, help break down complex foods, and synthesize certain vitamins. With so many useful (or 'friendly') organisms destroyed, yeast *(Candida albicans)* can grow unchecked, causing infections that have many troubling and seemingly unrelated symptoms, and which can cause or contribute to the leakiness of the gut. This unhealthy situation leads to more infections, more antibiotics and...well, you get the idea. (12)

Dr. Crook has, in the course of his long career, treated hundreds of autistic children. He has seen, over and over, the pattern described above. He has pioneered the use of low-sugar diets and anti-fungal medication, and many children have been helped significantly by his treatment. Despite the fact that the majority of mainstream medicine has scoffed at the notion of disease being caused by an organism that naturally occurs in our intestines, improvement is too widespread to dismiss and other doctors are now looking into the 'yeast connection.' (12)

Recent work by Dr. William Shaw, a Kansas City biochemist, is providing additional evidence to support Dr. Crook's long held theories. Shaw has found unusually high levels of fungal metabolites (yeast waste products) in the urine of several groups of abnormally functioning individuals, including people with autism. His first paper describing this phenomenon was published in 1995, and he is currently conducting further studies on the effect of anti-fungal therapy on urinary organic acids from children with autism. (57-59)

According to Dr. Stephen B. Edelson, as *Candida* proliferates in the gut it can undergo anatomical and physiological changes to become a different kind of fungus, a *mycelial fungus*. (18) *Candida's* original state is non-invasive, but as a mycelial fungus it produces structures which penetrate mucosal linings and break down the lining between the intestines and the rest of the circulation. In other words, *Candida* infections may also contribute to damage of the gut wall, enabling large molecules to cross the blood-brain barrier. Edelson points out that this damage could be introducing many substances into the blood which should not be there, and thus it is not surprising that many people with yeast overgrowth also show allergies to foods and environmental substances. Edelson cites work in England and in the U.S. at the National Institutes of Health that supports the notion that "some of these incomplete protein-breakdown products, if absorbed, may have endorphin-like activity and can change mood, mind, memory and behavior." (18)

Critics of the 'yeast connection' syndrome argue that not every illness can be cured by anti-fungal medication and special diets. This is certainly true. But it is also true that many people, adults as well as children, have been on an antibiotic 'merry-go-round' that has damaged their body's ability to heal itself and fight off infections. Anyone who has ever taken erythromycin or doxycycline can attest to the fact that it causes intense gastrointestinal discomfort. Why is it so difficult to accept that these medications do damage, in some people, that outlasts the course of the medication or the illness for which it was prescribed?

If you believe your health or your child's is compromised by an overgrowth of yeast, there are medical tests that can be performed (see Chapter 3). If these tests are positive, a course of one of the anti-fungal medications will probably be necessary. So too, will be a highly restrictive diet. However, many parents report significant improvements in their children's behavior as a result of this diet, and it is possible to follow the diet for the period generally required to improve health and behavior.

While I am not promoting the old saw "You are what you eat", mounting evidence suggests that dietary interventions are potentially helpful for a wide range of diseases and disorders. As unlikely as it may have sounded when you began this chapter, dietary intervention can truly help some children with autism, by removing allergens and biologically active peptides thereby reducing the load that an already over-taxed detoxification system must handle.

Chapter 3
Allergy or Intolerance?

Many children and adults claim to suffer from food **allergies**. While most physicians maintain that food allergies are extremely rare and food **sensitivity or intolerance** is non-existent, (4) in a vast number of cases these patients have found relief when treated with elimination and rotation diets. Although the incidence of this problem may have increased in the twentieth century, its existence was recorded in the time of Hippocrates, who noted that cow's milk could cause hives and stomach aches. "One man's meat is another man's poison" is believed to have been written by the Roman poet Lucretius, and the saying seems to be just as true today.

No one doubts that food allergies do exist; most people know someone for whom eating peanuts, or seafood would present a life-threatening situation. But negative reactions to food are far more widespread than are these deathly allergies. (13,38,40,44)

The term "allergy" has a specific, medical meaning, but it is often used inappropriately to describe a sensitivity or intolerance. According to the American Academy of Allergy and Immunology[1], food allergy can be defined as "any adverse reaction to an otherwise harmless food or food component that involves the body's immune system." Any substance that causes an immunological reaction is called an **allergen**, and the introduction of an allergen in a susceptible person causes **antibodies** to that allergen to be released. It is the release of the antibodies which trigger the allergic reaction.

The potential for developing food allergies is believed to be inherited; people with this genetic makeup produce increased amounts of IgE, a type of antibody produced by the immune system. When the immune system is stimulated by the ingestion of the food allergen, millions of these antibodies are produced and circulate throughout the body. Once they begin to circulate in the bloodstream, they bind to blood cells called **basophils**. As basophils they can enter body tissues and bind to **mast** cells. Mast cells are the immune system components responsible for producing many of the characteristic symptoms of allergies. Both basophils and mast cells produce various substances (e.g. histamine) which cause the unpleasant reactions we think of as allergy symptoms. (4,18,44)

In simplest terms, a food allergy is any negative reaction to an otherwise innocuous food or food component that involves the immune system. Allergy, in its strictest terms, involves *only* those food reactions that invoke this system.

The most common symptoms of true food allergies are stomach upset, vomiting, hives, eczema, headache, runny and/or stuffy nose, asthma and sometimes swelling of the lips or tongue. In rare, severe cases, the upper airway can swell, causing suffocation if medical help is not obtained within minutes. The foods most likely to cause food allergies, according to the American College of Allergy, Asthma and Immunology, are milk, fish, nuts, seafood, soy and wheat. Often, when one food is not tolerated, foods in the same botanical family also cause reactions (e.g. a person allergic to peanuts may not tolerate other legumes such as peas and beans).

According to Dr. Kazuhiko Kakuta, the rate of food allergy in the population of Japan has increased dramatically. (30) Kakuta claims that one in three Japanese suffer from some sort of allergy. He attributes this to the "deterioration of the living and dietary environment" that has triggered the growing number of skin, asthma and upper respiratory reactions in his patients. He believes that "...food is polluted by chemical substances...such as agrochemical and food additives. My suspicion is that the human body rejects the polluted food and produces allergy as a means of avoiding the risk of being harmed by polluted food." (30) Such pollutants may also be responsible for overloading the detoxification system, or for increasing the leakiness of the gut. (1)

As discussed in Chapter 1, middle ear infections are very prevalent in young children today. Antibiotics have been so heavily prescribed that most of the bacteria causing these infections have become resistant to the usual Amoxycillin treatment. Doctors are now prescribing more and more powerful and expensive drugs to treat these infections. (52) Many parents wonder why their children are plagued with these infections when they themselves managed to grow up without them.

Today, millions of children have these infections over and over in the first two to three years of their lives. Over half a million children per year end up with tubes surgically implanted in their ear drums to keep the fluid that forms from collecting and becoming infected. In fact, it is now estimated that 70.5% of all American infants have been given at least one course of antibiotics by the age of six months.[2]

A 1994 study indicates that food allergies may be at the root of many recurrent infections. In a study performed at the Georgetown University School of Medicine, Talal Nsouli and his colleagues performed food allergy testing on 104 children who had recurrent ear infections. Eighty-one of these children proved allergic to some foods, with a third of these children allergic to milk and another third allergic to wheat. Parents were instructed to keep the children off the offending foods for a period of four months. Seventy children improved, with significant clearing of the ear. Parents were then instructed to put the offending foods back into the diet of their children. Within four months, the ears were again clogged in sixty-six of the children! (38)

How do you know if your child has true (immune mediated) food allergies? The two most common types of test are skin prick tests and blood tests. In a skin prick test, a diluted extract of various foods (and other common allergens such as mold, pollens, dust, etc.) are placed on the skin, which is then scratched or pricked. If a red blimp or "wheal" appears within fifteen minutes, the test for the substance is considered positive and the person *may* be allergic to it. (44)

Two blood tests, the radioallergosorbent test (RAST) and the enzyme linked immunosorbent assay (ELISA), provide similar information. Neither test, however, is considered conclusive evidence of allergy. (44) When results are positive, an elimination diet is generally used to confirm the test results. Some doctors consider the elimination diet to be the only reliable means by which to diagnose food allergies accurately, and thus choose to skip skin and blood tests altogether.

In an *elimination diet*, suspected allergens are removed entirely from the diet, generally for a period of two to four weeks. If the person improves, the suspected foods are returned to the diet, one at a time, to see which foods cause a reaction and which are tolerated. If food allergies are confirmed by an elimination diet, the foods must be avoided entirely, or only tried occasionally, unless they produce life-threatening reactions (typical of peanut and seafood allergies). (13,44) Some common food allergies (such as to milk or egg) are often outgrown and there may come a time when they can be added back into the diet.

In some cases, a small amount of an allergic food does not provoke a reaction and these people can often follow *rotation diets*. A rotation diet brings variety, but it must be followed carefully to prevent troublesome foods from being eaten too often or in too large a quantity.

Because of the difficulty in determining exactly which component of a particular food is causing a problem, a child may seem allergic or intolerant to many foods. (18) For such children, some nutritionists suggest beginning with a selection of foods that are both unlikely to cause a reaction in anyone, and are completely novel to the child. Often such a rotation diet of very unusual foods results in significant improvement within a few weeks (if foods were indeed the source of the problems). At that point, more familiar foods may be added back to the diet, one at a time, to see whether or not they are tolerated. If an added food is tolerated at first, but then begins to cause symptoms, it is probably one that can be eaten only in moderation or on a rotational basis.

Unusual foods are hard to find and tend to be expensive, but a trial like this may result in a very positive response. Since more common foods are eventually allowed back into the diet, the expense will lessen over time. Karen Slimak is a nutritional consultant who began investigating unusual foods when her own children proved to have multiple food and environmental allergies. Mrs. Slimak worked to find unusual foods that could be processed into flours and other food ingredients. She later started a company that sells these unusual foods,[3] which contain no additives, preservatives, or added sugar.[4] (See Appendix I for more information.) Some of these products appear to be good additions for parents trying to follow "Sara's Diet," because they contain few pigments and add variability to a very restrictive regimen. Both rotation and elimination diets are covered extensively in books on the subject of food allergy (see, for example, Rapp's *Is This Your Child?*). (29)

If a true allergen is eaten, either as a test of the food or by accident, a reaction should occur. If this happens, doctors recommend several simple remedies to alleviate the symptoms.

The simplest is drinking a glass of water into which a teaspoon of unbuffered, powdered Vitamin C has been mixed. If this is not helpful, try Alka Seltzer® Gold (the non-aspirin form in a gold package).

Food intolerance is a more general term that refers to a negative reaction to a food that does not involve the immune system. (18) In these cases, the results of the skin and blood tests used in allergy testing will be negative.[5] Many times the cause of the intolerance is not known, but it is likely that many incoherences are the result of metabolic reaction. As explained in Chapter 2, genetic mutations can change the structure of an enzyme in a way that prevents it from digesting the protein it was intended to modify. There are thousands of enzymes devoted to the task of digestion and a deficiency in just one can cause serious problems.

One intolerance familiar to most people is the inability to digest lactose, the sugar in milk. *Lactose intolerance* occurs when there is insufficient lactase (an enzyme) to digest lactose. This results in gastrointestinal problems, which can be quite severe. Another well-known food intolerance is Celiac Disease. As discussed in Chapter 1, celiacs are not allergic to gluten but have a metabolic disorder that prevents it from being properly digested. There are no doubt many other metabolic reactions to food, in which the body cannot digest a particular food component.

S. A. Bock and F. M. Atkins (4) analyzed numerous studies that focused on food intolerance in children. They found that reactions to foods, while common, are generally caused by a relatively small number of foods. Ninety-five percent of all food intolerance reactions were found to be caused by **eggs, milk, nuts, soy, fish, corn and wheat**. It seems significant that the foods acknowledged as common causes of food reactions are the very same ones suspected to be causing problems for children with autism and multiple food sensitivities.

One of the reasons many doctors have insisted that food intolerance does not exist (except in very specific cases such as lactose intolerance) is that reactions to these foods may not be immediate.[6] In a delayed response, the reaction can occur anywhere from an hour to a day after eating the offending food. When a food allergy causes an immediate reaction it's fairly simple to isolate because these people usually react to only a few foods. Delayed responders, however, generally react to several foods, and often crave those foods which cause problems for them. This is rarely the case with true food allergies or immediate responders. (18)

Many parents are certain their children have food intolerances, but when they tell their doctors, the doctor prescribes an *allergy test*. When the test, predictably, is negative, what can be done? After all, we live in a society which respects and reveres medical doctors. But what do you do when your doctor dismisses your concern or worse yet, laughs at it? This kind of reaction probably explains why parents of children on the autistic spectrum give up the notion of the all-knowing doctor in fairly short order. This was stated very succinctly by autism expert Dr. Lorna Wing, in her foreword to the Bryna Siegel book *The World of the Autistic Child*. Wing writes: "Parents of children with autistic spectrum disorders. . .do not, in general, have a high opinion of professionals." (1996.)

I must admit to laughing out loud at the understatement of this sentence. When parents come upon, either by dint of hard research or by accident, something that does help their child, many doctors often dismiss the idea as silly. This is the most common reaction parents meet if they decide to bring up dietary interventions with their physicians. In the last three years, I have received countless letters from parents stating that the diet has genuinely helped their child but their doctor will not believe it in the absence of double blind experiments published in medical journals.

There are *some* doctors who believe and accept parent observations of their young patients, but if you have no such doctor to help you, do not become discouraged. If you've seen positive changes—great. But if you have yet to begin a dietary trial, keep in mind the skepticism of doctors, grandparents, teachers and sitters. One to two weeks before starting any dietary changes, take baseline data on your child's behavior. Baseline data is usually presented graphically. If done well, it can function as a 'Before Picture' of sorts. Data which notes the frequency and/or duration of specific behaviors (see chart A) establishes a picture of the pre-diet behavior, and gives you objective information which can be used for comparison with post-diet data.

Once you begin changing the diet, be sure to continue collecting data for as long as you can, preferable for a few months. (see chart B) Note every time the diet or other factors (e.g. new vitamins or medication) have changed. Be scrupulous about your data collection and get others to help when they are watching your son or daughter. Make many copies of the chart, and be careful to record the dates. If at all possible, follow the scientific method—change only one thing at a time so you do not confuse your results. If other changes occur, e.g. self-training for the toilet, the sudden improvement in language or cognitive ability, note these changes too.[7] Since many of these kids also experience bowel difficulties, be sure to note frequency and consistency of movements, and note any changes from the usual pattern. It may be possible to have data takers (teachers or therapists, for example) who are "blind" to the diet. That is, if they are not told what foods are being excluded or when the trials begin, they will collect data more objectively. This may not always be possible, but if you are providing all foods for meals and snacks, you may be able to collect data from people who are truly blind to the start (and possibly the end) of a dietary intervention.

This type of data collection is a reasonably objective means by which to show behavioral changes. While this system may not be as conclusive as double-blind, placebo controlled studies, most doctors will accept changes they see in black and white. If your child suffers a withdrawal type of response, keep taking data and stay with the diet! You may see an immediate increase in problem behaviors followed, generally within 1-3 weeks, by a steady improvement.

What else should concern parents about our children's diets? When the Feingold diet first came to public attention, many parents rushed to remove all artificial colors and flavors, as well as all *food additives*. Should we worry about these additives? Will this not make it even harder to keep your child eating the right foods? Alas, the answer to both questions is probably yes. Recall however, that fresh or minimally processed foods are generally allowed on this diet, and have very few additives. Since most breads and other baked goods are likely homemade or purchased in a natural foods store, they too should be additive-free.

Additives have been used to preserve food for hundreds of years, but it was only in the last fifty years that companies began using multiple and questionable additives meant to preserve the shelf life of foods for very extended periods. In the sixties, Americans began to buy convenience foods in increasing quantities. The artificial additives that went into these foods were viewed as advancements, and people accepted such slogans as "Better living through chemistry" without a second thought.

Farmers began using newly developed chemicals to preserve fresh produce, allowing it to arrive at market with minimal spoilage. They routinely spray fruits and vegetables with harmful pesticides and ripening agents, most of which are extremely hard to wash off.

Recently, there has been heated debate about whether farmers should be allowed to give their dairy cattle hormones to increase the production of milk. In addition to questions about the safety of milk from such cows, many people believe it is cruel to the cow.[8]

The Food and Drug Administration (FDA) is the governmental organization responsible for determining the safety of food additives. A popular label that is applied to many of these additives is GRAS (Generally Regarded As Safe). GRAS items include those additives that are widely used and believed to be safe enough to be exempt from further testing. At first, many GRAS items were actually poorly tested. Many food additives eventually had their GRAS rating removed with a subsequent banning of the additives (e.g. the cyclamates which gave Americana their first good tasting diet sodas, met this fate). (34)

Standards required to earn the GRAS label are generally higher than they were twenty years ago. But even with stricter standards, the FDA is not infallible. There is little doubt that many additives "generally regarded as safe" today will ultimately be found to be unhealthful at the very least, and some may actually be toxic to humans. In general, it is safest to avoid additives as much as possible. There are many however, which really are safe and do not need to be avoided. A list of some of the most common additives and their relative safety follows.

SAFE ADDITIVES

Acacia Gum

Adenosine 5 (avoid on yeast-free diet)

Adipic Acid

Caselnates (avoid on CF diet)

Ammonium Salt Compounds

Annatto Color (avoided by *some* celiacs)

Ascorbic Acid

Ascorbyl Palmitate

Beta Carotene (avoid on "white diets")

Calcium Ascorbate, phosphate, salts, sulfate

Carbonates

Cellulose gel, gum

Disodium Inosinate (avoid in yeast-free diets)

EDTA

Fumaric Acid

Gelatin

Glycerides

Lactic acid (avoid if very sensitive to dairy)

Lecithin (avoid if soy is a problem)

Pectin

Potassium chloride, citrate, phosphate, sorbate

Psyllium

Xanthan gum

AVOID THESE ADDITIVES

All aluminum compounds

Artificial colors

Artificial flavors

Aspartame (Nutrasweet)

BHA

BHT

Caffeine

Calcium Disodium EDTA

FD&C colors

Monosodium Glutamate (MSG)

Nitrates

Nitrites

Phosphoric acid

Potassium Bromate

Quinine

Olestra

Polysorbate 60, 80

Saccharin

Sulfites

Vanillin (common artificial flavor)

TBHQ

Source: *The Label Reader's Pocket Dictionary of Food Additives* (1993). J. Michael Lapchick with Cindy Appleseth, R.Ph. Chronomed Publishing: Minneapolis, MN.

Chart A

PRE-DIET "BASELINE" DATA COLLECTION SHEET

Date:_____

Food Eaten: _____

Time Eaten: _____

Behavior & Time it Occured: _____

_____

Food Eaten: _____

Time Eaten: _____

Behavior & Time it Occured: _____

_____

Food Eaten: _____

Time Eaten: _____

Behavior & Time it Occured: _____

_____

Comments: Note anything unusual or odd in the child's behavior (either positive or negative). Note anything at all here, even if you don't think it is significant. You may later be able to see a pattern, when comparing sheets from many days.

If your child has a history of bowel problems you should also make a note of bowel frequency and character.

Chart B

BEHAVIOR CHART POST-DIETARY IMPLEMENTATION

Types of behaviors are listed. Use any that your child regularly performs.

Date:_____

BEHAVIOR	FREQUENCY	DURATION
	(record # of occurrences)	(record in increments of 1-5 minutes)

Responsiveness

Uses toilet

Tantrums

Hand/Finger play

Aggression, SIB

Head Banging

Self-stimulatory behaviors

Spinning toys

Giddiness

Verbalizes needs

Screaming

Noncompliance

Other

COMMENTS: Make the same kind of notations as suggested on Chart A. For behaviors that occur in discrete increments, such as spinning a toy, record the number of separate instances of the behavior. For behaviors such as tantrums, record the duration of the episode.

NOTES

Chapter 4
Tests and Nutritional Supports

When parents first receive a diagnosis of autism for their child, it is difficult for them to know what steps they need to take. Very few parents have any experience that prepares them for what lies ahead. It is hard to believe that one's child has such a pervasive problem to begin with, but perhaps harder to accept is the fact that the medical profession has so little to offer. When our child received this diagnosis in 1991, many professionals told us that we were 'lucky' because, in the past, autism was more a sentence than a diagnosis. We were also led to believe that while doctors had little to offer, the educational system held great promise.

We immediately began to do research and what we found wasn't all that encouraging. It was true that educators were showing some good results using applied behavior analysis (ABA) techniques such as those pioneered by Lovaas, and it was also true that the area in which we live has several excellent schools for autistic children. But miracles weren't exactly happening, and we were stunned to learn how few medical tests were done, and how little research had been undertaken. It did not seem likely that much research would be done in the near future either, once we found out just how few research dollars were being allocated to autism.

Such funding for autism research provided little incentive for bright young scientists to devote themselves to this particular disorder. Another problem is that autism is a very nebulous diagnosis. It was realized long ago that many different etiologies (causes) might account for the same set (or subset) of symptoms. The way in which the diagnosis is made illustrates this point quite well-there is no known medical test that can positively identify autism in a child. So far, there is no test to show damage to particular genes, no one inborn error of metabolism that unequivocally shows that a child has autism. The diagnosis is based on behavioral grounds, usually by someone familiar with the DSM-IV description of autistic symptoms.

There is not a single drug currently approved by the FDA for autism; that does not mean drugs are not prescribed. Doctors do prescribe medication to address particular symptoms of the disorder, such as attention deficits, hyperactivity and aggression. All of the medications used, however, were created for and approved for use in other diseases and disorders. While medicines benefit some autistics, none address the underlying physiological causes. Few are without the potential for side effects, some of which can be very serious.

Several years ago, the late Dr. Roland Ciaranello of Stanford University was asked (on an Internet forum) why there wasn't much research money being dedicated to autism. Ciaranello had devoted years to autism research, setting up a large scale, multi-family gene study. Many parents took offense when he suggested that parents had at least a share of the blame. He pointed out that in nearly every other disease or disorder, parents had organized and lobbied for funding, bringing it into public awareness and finding political allies who could be enlisted to help. Perhaps the overwhelming strain that autism puts on a family made such organization seem impossible. The Autism Society of America has been in existence for nearly thirty years, but they have focused on support for families and education for the public. While worthwhile goals, the ASA has only recently begun to focus on research in autism.

It wasn't until 1967 that the medical profession (at least in the U.S.) dropped the idea that autism was a psychogenic disorder caused by "refrigerator mothers," to use Bruno Bettleheim's designation. Dr. Bernard Rimland published the book that once and for all showed that autism has a biological cause, and it was Rimland who, along with other parents, started the National Society for Autistic Children (NSAC) which later evolved into the ASA. Rimland also runs Autism Research Institute, an organization devoted to following autism research and keeping parents informed.[1]

Realizing how little was really being done in autism research, a few years ago Rimland invited a select group of scientists to attend a workshop and define needed research and treatment goals. Calling his effort "Defeat Autism Now!" the first meeting took place in Dallas in 1995.[2] Over the course of three days, a set of promising research directions were outlined. However, since an important goal of the DAN! group was to give parents and physicians ideas for treatment options now, a major topic of discussion surrounded what tests could be done to determine if particular available treatments were suitable for particular children.

While researchers in attendance did not always agree on the relative importance of every research avenue explored, in general this first meeting was extremely useful.[3] Everyone present agreed that guidance for parents and doctors was desperately needed. Two group members, Drs. Sidney Baker and Jon Pangborn, offered to work together to write a research protocol based on the discussions that took place. It was published under the title "Biomedical Assessment Options for Children with Autism and Related Problems." The Dan! Protocol, as it has come to be known, is available for $25 from the Autism Research Institute.[4]

I would strongly urge readers to obtain a copy of the protocol, and find a doctor who will review it with you and help you determine which of the outlined tests seem worth doing, based on the symptoms your child exhibits. The protocol clearly defines every included test, the rationale for performing it, as well as listing the routine tests that should have been performed during initial diagnosis. It is not my intention to cover the same ground here, but I would like to discuss a few of the tests most appropriate to consider prior to committing your child and entire family to a dietary intervention.

When I removed dairy, and later gluten from my son's diet, I did so without having performed any tests which would have indicated a need or even a probability of efficacy. I was merely exploring anything that might prove helpful, and I suppose I got lucky. When I later did some research on the topic, I realized that there were some tests which probably should have been done. I chose not to do them, however, because Sum had been on a gluten-free diet for a very long time and had already shown great improvement. I was unwilling to start over, purposely feeding him foods that I believed were harmful to him.

In retrospect, I wish I had done more testing before starting the diet. However, since Sam ate a wide variety of foods, and accepted his new diet so easily, trying this intervention had really presented no problems for us. Since that time I have heard from so many parents whose children eat a very limited diet and are extremely resistant to trying anything new. Making a radical dietary change will be very traumatic for these families, and it is just common sense to determine whether a GF/CF diet is likely to help before proceeding.

Before you start, you should realize that very few tests are totally reliable—all give some percentage of false positive or negative results. For this reason it is important that you work with a doctor who is knowledgeable about autism *and* these tests. If your child's symptoms clearly indicate to the physician that a particular treatment might help but test results show otherwise, you might want to discuss his reasoning and try the treatment anyway. Unless the suggested treatment is potentially harmful, this would be a good approach to follow *if you trust that your doctor 's opinions are reasonable based on his or her knowledge and, perhaps more important, experience.*

Urine and Blood Tests

There is no definitive test that will tell you that a GF/CF diet will help your child, or how much it might help. There is a test, however, which will show whether the child's urine shows the characteristic peaks seen in the research described in Chapter 1. Reichelt and his colleagues in Norway have found a close association between the presence of the peaks and improvement on a GF/CF diet. Shattock's group is undertaking a similar test of the diet.[5] In this country, many parents have sent samples to Dr. Robert Cade at the University of Florida at Gainesville. Directions for the collection and shipment of the specimen can be obtained by calling Dr. Cade's assistant, Malcom Privette, at 352-392-8952.

The urine test is free, but an associated blood test is performed by a commercial laboratory at a charge of $64. Actually, this is a panel of tests run on a single sample, in which blood serum is assayed for IgA and IgG antibodies to the following proteins: gliadin, gluten, lactalbumin, beta-lactoglobulin, casein and ovalbumin. It is convenient that Dr. Cade's lab is in the United States of course, and it is helpful that there is no charge for the urine testing. The disadvantage however, is that Dr. Cade requires a 24-hour urine collection, even though it has been determined that a single, first morning sample is sufficient for accurate testing. Because Dr. Cade's early tests were all performed on 24-hour samples, he continues to use this sampling technique to maintain the integrity of his data. For children who are not toilet trained, however, getting 24 hours worth of urine is very difficult to accomplish.

Dr. Reichelt will also test urine for the presence of abnormal peptides, but asks that the patient obtain the collection kit and directions from a doctor (participating doctors are listed in the DAN! protocol). Doctors typically stockpile samples in the freezer until they have several; then they are shipped to Dr. Reichelt's lab in Norway. Dr. Reichelt also requires blood testing; blood is collected by your doctor and sent to Alletess Medical in Rockland, MD for analysis.

Positive tests of the blood and/or urine samples certainly argue strongly for the implementation of the GF/CF diet. If the possibility of trying this diet is particularly daunting, you may wish to wait until you receive the results. Be warned, however, that parents report delays of up to six months for receiving test results! If a child will benefit from the diet, the earlier it is implemented the better. Therefore, it probably makes sense to begin a gradual dietary change (see discussion in Chapter 5) as soon as the urine and blood samples have been collected for these tests, and those for **Celiac Disease** (see next section.) This way, no time is lost. Should results turn out to be negative, you can always reintroduce any foods you have removed. For the most part, the diet is probably more healthful than what many children eat currently, and it is unlikely to hurt them in any way.

Tests for Celiac Disease

While they are not part of the DAN! Protocol, blood tests are available which can show latent and sub-clinical cases of Celiac Disease. According to pediatric gastroenterologist Dr. Karoly Horvath[6], blood tests exist which have a greater than 90% sensitivity and specificity to exclude celiac disease *prior to starting a gluten-free diet*. This should certainly be done if the child has a history of chronic loose stools, since chronic diarrhea is a known manifestation of Celiac Disease. Because even latent celiac disease will cause damage to the intestinal wall, it is reasonable to run these tests even in the absence of chronic bowel symptoms.

Most people will be able to obtain insurance coverage for such tests, particularly if there is a history of gastrointestinal symptoms. The relevant tests involve screening the blood for celiac antibodies. The tests are called **endomysial IgA, gliadin IgA and reticulin IgA**. The blood test can rule out or suggest Celiac Disease.[7]

While these tests *will not* reveal a possible sensitivity to casein, they should certainly be done on children who developed normally up to two years (and who are thus more likely sensitive to gluten), in addition to those with a history of chronic bowel problems. Not all laboratories are equipped to run these tests. If your doctor is unable to find a local source, suggest that he or she contact Specialty Laboratories, Inc., Santa Monica, CA at 310-828-6543.

Although no child will willingly donate blood, all four tests can be performed following a single draw. It is not my intention to suggest that all autistic people will turn out to have celiac disease, but the tests should be performed to rule it out. Certainly CD causes a leaky gut; if various proteins are being improperly metabolized, such a gut would provide a pathway into the bloodstream for these peptides. These tests should probably be added to the battery that children undergo when a diagnosis of autism, PDD-NOS or atypical autism is first made.

Gut Permeability

As discussed in Chapter 1, an increased permeability of the gut wall allows peptides, microbial organic acids (see below) and other substances to enter the bloodstream.(6,14) This permeability can be caused by many things, including a PST deficiency and imbalances in the intestinal flora, the bacteria that are normal residents of your gut.(56) There is a test of gut permeability (also called a "leaky gut test") which is based on the differential absorption of two distinct sugars.[8] This test is also part of the DAN! Protocol, where it is described more fully.

It is not clear whether removal of the offending proteins actually allows the gut to heal, or whether it remains permeable, but biologically active proteins are no longer present to pass through to the bloodstream. Healing the gut takes time, and there is considerable disagreement on whether any products currently available are really helpful. Some professionals believe you must remove offending foods and then just wait. Others maintain that certain herbs and nutrients may help heal the gut (e.g. slippery elm, aloe vera drinks or supplements, and Fructooligo-saccharides).

Detoxification Tests

Dr. Waring's finding that autistic children often have a weakness in the PST system has sparked a great deal of interest in tests which reveal weakness in this and other detoxification pathways. Dr. Waring has tested urine samples in the past, but does not currently have the resources to do large scale testing. In America, this test is analyzed, again, by the Great Smokies Diagnostic Laboratories. When a doctor orders the test, generally referred to as a "Liver Detoxification Test," you will receive instructions and materials for collecting a 24-hour urine sample. The test uses a chemical 'probe' to measure the body's efficiency in detoxification. The probe consists of acetaminophen (Tylenol®), caffeine and aspirin (all given in small, safe doses.)

Another detoxification test, **MHPG sulfate and glucuronide ratios**, is performed by SmithKline Beecham Laboratories. (See Ref.60 for a detailed explanation.) Which of the two tests gives the best indication of detoxification efficiency is unclear at this time, but some may prefer this test because it does not require the use of the chemical probe.

If detoxification pathways are found to be deficient, diet can be used to reduce the toxic load, and nutritional supplements may again be useful. Foods known to cause problems for individuals with deficient PST include chocolate, bananas and oranges. (39, 65) Vitamins C and E may be useful, and doctors may suggest amino acids such as reduced L-glutathione and N-acetylcysteine. (17) Antioxidants such as selenium and bioflavonoids are valuable for detoxification in general, and the herb Milkweed Thistle is reputedly helpful for liver detoxification. (36) You should not attempt to supplement amino acids without the advice of a knowledgeable doctor or nutritionist, preferably one who is well-versed in alternative medical treatments.

Organic Acids

Organic acids are normal metabolic substances that can appear in the tissues, blood and urine in abnormal amounts when a metabolic error prevents normal metabolism or detoxification. Traditional organic acid tests have been used for years to identify a few severe metabolic errors (e.g. PKU). Recently, Dr. William Shaw identified children with significant developmental delays who excreted very large amounts of some of these acids.(57)

Dr. Shaw identified these organic acids as the byproducts of fungi and bacteria. He has devised a test that will indicate whether you need to make further changes to your child's diet and if an anti-fungal or anti-bacterial medication is in order. (12) Levels of the harmful organic acids drop when appropriate medication is used, and Dr. Shaw believes that if suitable measures are taken when indicated, the child will show much improvement. The test requires a urine sample, and is performed by Dr. Shaw's laboratory, The Great Plains Laboratory for Health, Metabolism and Nutrition. (http://www.autism.com/shaw-yeast/contents.html#toc or call 913-341-8949). You will be sent a test kit with directions for the collection and shipping of the sample. The test costs $200, but Dr. Shaw has good advice on getting your insurance to cover it. Be sure to ask about insurance company pointers when you call the lab for a test kit.

After The Tests...What To Do Next

It is important to remember to try only one new intervention at a time. Often parents take the attitude that they will try several things at once, stating "I don't care which thing is helping...he is better!" This kind of approach could very well lead to months or even years of unnecessary medication or adherence to a very limited diet. If one thing seems to help 'a little' you might be tempted to add an additional treatment. Perhaps the combination of two therapies will really help a lot, or perhaps it might cause a negative response. What will this tell you? Does it mean that the second agent is causing harm? Does it mean that the second agent should be stopped immediately? It might, but it could also be that the second intervention might have been far more useful than the first, but that the two cannot be combined. It is safer to try the two separately and assess the effects of each. Once done, you can try a combination. If there is a negative reaction you will be able to decide which of the two agents gave the most benefit when used alone. **(Remember, NEVER combine medications without checking with your doctor to ensure that such a combination is safe!)**

If you go ahead and have the above tests performed, while you wait for results try B_6 and magnesium supplementation, if you haven't already done so. There is a great deal of information available (43) to indicate that such a trial is safe, and for many people, very effective. This would also be a good time to try DMG, although you should see the effects of the B_6 therapy first before adding a second supplement. For some children, DMG seems almost miraculous—for others, no reaction is observed at all. Try to record the frequency and duration of problem behaviors, and note other problems such as "won't sleep" or "extreme hyperactivity" prior to beginning this supplementation. After beginning the trial, record dosages and take similar data to compare with the pre-supplement information.

Also while you wait for test results, begin the process of weaning your child off cow's milk. You might start by trying various non-dairy beverages (see Appendix II) to determine which look and taste the best to your family. When you find one that works (make sure it is also GF) begin the process of mixing small amounts of it in with real milk, gradually increasing the amount of substitute being used. Remember, you can always return to dairy if all tests are negative. Many companies will send you a free sample of their product. Do not be afraid to ask.

You might also begin to experiment with some GF foods, adding them into the diet long before you remove the old foods. If your child is a juice addict, at this time begin to water down juices and substitute pear for apple (baby pear juice looks and tastes just like apple juice). White grape juice is also fairly innocuous—introduce it in a watered down form and in very small amounts. Again, should the tests come back negative, or should you decide you do not want to try this diet, you can always go back to previous food choices.

You can also begin to reduce sugar in your family's diet. Many times you can simply reduce the amount of sweetener used, and you can begin to shop for foods that have fewer additives, hydrogenated or partially hydrogenated oils and artificial colors and flavors. Cook whole grains instead of serving only processed or refined ones. Choose brown rice instead of white. If a fruit or vegetable cannot be peeled or scrubbed prior to eating, choose organic sources. Think about planting a garden if space permits—if you grow and pick it yourself, you know exactly what did (or didn't) get put on the plants.

Begin baking non-yeast (quick) breads or try a few of the GF bread mixes so widely available. Visit a health food store—you will be amazed at what you will find there. Most important of all, begin to read food labels. REALLY read them and understand what they mean—if you don't understand them (and some are nearly incomprehensible) ask questions. If you have Internet access (which I strongly urge you to get) begin to visit consumer advocacy and other informational web sites (see Appendix IV). If you don't have a computer, visit your local library—in addition to print resources, most libraries have Internet connected computers available for your use, and librarians trained to help you. If you use this waiting time well, you will be ready to begin the diet full scale if the tests come back positive.

Once you decide to try diet or any other intervention, you must learn to be patient. It helps to set up a predetermined trial period and stay with it before abandoning the intervention. Just as some medications can take a long time to build up to a therapeutic blood level, diets and other supplements vary. It is unfortunate, but true, that diets generally take time to show their effects. This has led many parents to abandon a trial too quickly.

In England, Shattock's group has observed that when very small children are put on a GF/CF diet cold turkey, they often experience severe withdrawal reactions. (One small child's reaction was so extreme that hospitalization was required.) This observation, coupled with the knowledge that the effects of gluten peptides stay in the system for a very long time,[9] led Shattock to theorize that older children and adults have much larger stores of these peptides than do small children. When gluten is suddenly removed, the stored opioids cause a gradual weaning until the excess in the system has been depleted. For very small children who have eaten these foods for a relatively short period, the stores are depleted so quickly that the sudden removal causes a strong withdrawal. Shattock's group now recommends a gradual removal of the offending proteins for children under the age of four.

One way to accomplish this gradual process is to remove all dairy for a few weeks, followed by the removal of all wheat.[10] After a few weeks, oats (and products that contain them) can be eliminated too. Finally, after a few more weeks, the removal of rye and barley results in a totally GF diet. For older children, this conservative approach probably isn't needed, but certainly wouldn't hurt.

Supplementation

There are many vitamin, mineral, amino acid and herb supplements that may be helpful to your child. Some of these are not recommended unless tests show deficiencies, but others are often tried simply because they are known to be safe and may affect your child's symptoms. It is vital that you work with a doctor or nutritionist who is very well versed with the treatment of autistic children and alternative therapies. The

DAN! Protocol is a good place to begin looking for such practitioners. Other parents are also good sources of professionals in your area.

The information presented below is widely available in encyclopedias and books about nutrition. It is a compilation of information taken from various sources, including books and articles (1,7,12,17-19, 23,36, 37, 49, 52), lectures I have attended and personal communication with doctors, nutritionists and other parents.

The information is not intended to be medical advice— it is for your evaluation and you should share it with your doctor or nutritionist.

Vitamins and Minerals

SupraNuThera (SNT)

This supplement compound consists primarily of a megadose of vitamin B-6 with magnesium, and was developed by Dr. Bernard Rimland. It includes additional vitamins and minerals that assist in the absorption and utilization of B-6. Many parents have used this product and noted various improvements in behavior, sleep patterns, speech and other behaviors. Some parents have not noted any changes. Side effects of diarrhea, rash or hyperactivity are generally transitory. Available from Kirkman Sales (800-245-8282), it comes in a powder or capsule form. Recently, Kirkman announced that SNT is available in a liquid form. Since it is difficult to give the compound to small children, it is expected that this new formulation will make it possible for many more parents to try the supplement. When taking SNT, other vitamins are unnecessary, although some mineral supplementation may be advised by your physician. Note that SNT does contain copper; if your child has tested as deficient in zinc, you will want to take a vitamin without copper, and add additional zinc (determine mineral levels in consultation with your doctor).

DiMethylGlycine (DMG)

This supplement, considered to be a food substance, is available in health food stores. It has had varying effects on children who have taken it. Reports from parents range from miraculous ("He began to talk the next day!") to "No effect whatsoever." Some children become quite hyperactive on DMG, but adding a folic acid supplement generally helps. Buy tablets wrapped in foil.

Vitamin A

Supports the immune system; generally taken in the form of beta carotene.

Vitamin B complex

If taking SNT, do not supplement with addition B vitamins. In general, the B vitamins aid in the digestion of fats and carbohydrates, promote nervous system normalcy, improve concentration, memory, balance, and support the immune system.

Vitamin C

Supports the immune system; it has anti-viral and anti-bacterial properties and reduces the effects of many allergy producing substances.

Citrus Bioflavonoids

Bioflavonoids are antioxidants that increase capillary strength and work with Vitamin C to keep connective tissue healthy. Bioflavonoids build resistance to infection. One bioflavonoid is called Pcynogenol. It is extracted from Pine Bark and grape seeds. Pcynogenol acts as a natural antibiotic.

Choline

Actually a B-complex member, some parents supplement with choline even if on SNT or another good B-6/magnesium combination. It emulsifies fats (and works best with inositol, another B-complex component) and reduces cholesterol. Choline can cross the blood-brain barrier. It has a soothing effect and increases memory and learning abilities. Can assist in detoxification by aiding the liver.

Calcium

Calcium works with phosphorus to promote healthy bones and teeth. It quickens reflexes by aiding the nervous system in impulse transmission. It should be taken in balance with magnesium, with approximately twice as much calcium as magnesium. Since the best source (dairy products) is avoided on this diet, other sources should be used. Calcium can be found in soybeans, sardines, salmon, peanuts, dried beans, tofu and green vegetables. Kirkman Labs makes an excellent calcium supplement. (phone: 1-800-245-8282, website: www.kirkmanlabs.com) Most calcium supplements also include Vitamin D, which is necessary for the proper absorption of calcium.

Vitamin E

While the jury is still out on Vitamin E supplementation, it is an active antioxidant. It should be taken with B complex, inositol and Vitamin C.

Folic Acid

Another B complex vitamin, folic acid is needed to utilize sugar and amino acids. Helps in the metabolism of protein and is needed for cell division.

Inositol

An important nutrient for brain cells, inositol is essential for the metabolism of fats. When combined with choline, lecithin is formed. Many people supplement with lecithin granules, adding them to baked foods or to drinks.

Magnesium

Magnesium is sometimes called the tranquility mineral, as it can decrease stress. It is necessary for calcium and vitamin C metabolism. While SNT or a calcium-magnesium supplement provides enough magnesium, a small amount of magnesium dissolved in water or juice may calm an excited child.

Molybdenum

A trace mineral that aids in carbohydrate and fat metabolism, molybdenum is often recommended for people with a known or suspected PST deficiency, or for people (e.g. asthmatics) who react negatively to sulfites added to foods.

Selenium

This antioxidant is often recommended for people on wheat-free diets, since wheat is the most common source. It Is believed to increase the activity of natural killer cells, and thus supports the immune system.

Zinc

Many children with autism measure very low in zinc. This important mineral is responsible for the maintenance of various enzyme systems and is necessary for protein synthesis. It has been found to be important in brain function. It can improve learning by increasing mental alertness.

Other Supplements

Amino Acids

Many doctors have suggested various amino acid supplements for their autistic patients, generally after testing has been done to uncover deficiencies. Some of these include L-methionine, L-taurine, L-lysine and Reduced L-Glutathione and are believed to help in the detoxification process. L-glutamine is important for gut barrier function; experimentally induced glutamine deficiency causes diarrhea and ulcers of the gut lining. Some studies indicate that glutamine and epidermal growth factor (a polypeptide) work together in thickening the small intestine.

Bacterial Innoculants

Some practitioners recommend 'good bacteria' when there is evidence of a yeast overgrowth. This is generally done along with a prescription for anti-fungal medication, but it is safe to take before, after and during anti-fungal treatment. The most common types are *Lactobacillus acidophilus and L. Bifidus.* Be certain to get a non-dairy version.

Essential Fatty Acids

EFAs are the chemical building blocks of fat, and are 'essential' because the body cannot make them. They are divided into two groups, the Omega 6 fats and the Omega 3s. Because they are present in many oils (e.g. sunflower and corn) most people do get enough Omega 6s. Omega 3s, however, are generally deficient in our diets. Furthermore, nearly every processed food we eat contains trans fats (hydrogenated or partially hydrogenated oils). Trans fats prevent the body from properly using EFAs and should be avoided whenever possible. The preservatives BHA and BHT and artificial colors and flavors also inhibit the conversion of EFAs to prostaglandins. Omega 3 fats can be obtained by supplementing with flax seed or flax seed oil, evening primrose oil, borage oil, fish oils and black currant seed oil. EFAs are critical to the immune system.

Fructooligosaccharides (FOS)

FOS are naturally occurring carbohydrates which, unlike other carbohydrates, are not absorbed in the upper gastrointestinal tract. Instead they are passed to the colon (undigested) where they can be fermented and used by the flora of the colon. FOS are used by the so-called 'friendly' bacteria e.g. Lactobacilli and Bifidobacteria. When these bacteria grow and reproduce, they suppress the growth of disease-causing bacteria and fungi.

MCT Oil

Medium Chain Triglyceride Oil is derived from coconut, and seems to have anti-viral, anti-fungal and antibacterial properties. MCT oil is a source of two medium chain fatty acids: caprylic acid and capric acid. It is absorbed directly into the blood, bypassing the lymphatic system, which may be significant in cases of improper intestinal function. Some nutritionists suggest a trial of MCT oil along with L-Carnitine.

L-Carnitine

L-Carnitine is essential for the metabolism of fats. It functions as a carrier of energy resources to neurons and assists in removing toxic by-products of brain metabolism.

Digestive Enzymes

Digestive enzymes derived from plants, notably papain (from papaya) and bromelain (from pineapple) are often given to facilitate the break-down of foods. Many doctors believe they are not strong enough to really help, and suggest a prescription enzyme. Do not use enzymes stronger than papain or bromelain for children who cannot swallow enterically coated pills (a coating that prevents damage to the mouth tissues and the breakdown of the enzyme in the acidic environment of the stomach).

Herbs & Botanicals

Natural Antibiotics:

Astragalus

A Chinese herb used for centuries, astragalus promotes resistance to disease and may restore normal immune function in people undergoing cancer treatments.

Black walnut

Black walnut is an anti-fungal and anti-parasitic herb. It also appears helpful in fighting off bacterial infections.

Echinacea

Derived from the American Cone Flower, echinacea is used in large amounts for short periods, generally when the first symptoms of a cold or flu appear. It increases the natural release of anti-viral substances. It should not be used long term, or it will lose its effectiveness.

Garlic

In addition to preventing heart disease by reducing blood pressure and blood lipids, garlic has anti-fungal properties. It has been shown to improve learning and memory in animal models. Supports the immune system.

Other Herbs:

Ginko Biloba

Ginko has been used for hundreds of years, and is believed to combat memory problems, tinnitus, headaches, and dizziness. It increases blood flow to the brain, improves cerebral metabolism, and reduces free-radical activity. Improves mental functioning and the ability to concentrate.

Gotu Kola

Gotu Kola may improve memory and brain function due to its beneficial effect on circulation. This herb has a calming effect on the body.

Milk Thistle

This herb contains the flavonoid silymarin and has a direct effect on the liver. It is believed to aid in detoxification.

Passionflower

This is a natural tranquilizer, which relieves muscle tension and anxiety. It is a safe way to induce relaxation, and when used with herbs such as hops and valerian, may cure insomnia. It is often combined with these and other herbs in tea, but can also be taken in drops mixed into a drink.

Pau d'Arco

Pau d'Arco is an old remedy for Candida, athlete's foot and other fungal infections. It reputedly helps to burst yeast cells and hinder their reproduction, helps fight parasitic infections and lowers blood sugar.

When buying herbs or herbal extracts, be aware that the producers are not closely regulated. Do research to determine which brands use the purest herbs and the most carefully quantified potency measurements. If your doctor suggests supplementation with vitamins, minerals or amino acids, be sure to buy brands that are free of additives and excipients. These are used as fillers and binding agents, and in general the cheaper the supplement, the more fillers you will find. In addition to avoiding vitamins and minerals which contain glucose, lactose, starch (unspecified), gluten or yeast, watch for these additives:

Propylene glycol

Sodium laurel sulfate

Sodium laureth sulfate

Sodium benzoate

BHT

BHA

Tartrazine

Magnesium stearate

Red dyes

Chapter 5
How (and What) to Feed
Your Child

Getting Started

I often hear from parents whose children eat only four foods, typically Chicken McNuggets®, french fries, pizza and milk. You may find it difficult to believe, but a GF/CF diet is possible for such a child. While real McNuggets® may be out, this is not an insurmountable problem, because, as you will see in Chapter 7, they are simple to make at home. Pizza is also possible, using non-wheat crusts and a mock cheese (see Chapter 7 for ideas.) Cow's milk must be eliminated, but there are many delicious alternatives[1] that have been accepted by even the pickiest of children (see Appendix III).

Dairy First

Because it is generally easier to eliminate all dairy products from the diet than to remove all traces of gluten, many people decide to eliminate dairy first, then gluten later. There are many milk substitutes, but be sure that you choose one that is also gluten-free. Even if you attempt to make this a gradual change, it makes no sense to have your child adjust to a substitute that will not be used later.

Soy 'milks' are easy to find and many are acceptable. Be aware, however, that many children are also allergic or sensitive to soy, so you may wish to try a rice or potato-based milk product. Many of these beverages come in powdered or liquid form—although the liquid is more convenient for drinking, you will want to have powder on hand too. Many of the gluten-free bread recipes (e.g. nearly all those in the Hagman books) call for powdered milk. Dry milk powder is also easy to use in recipes that call for liquid milk. For every cup of milk in the recipe, add 8 oz. of water to the wet ingredients, and 2-3 TBL. dry milk powder to the dry ingredients. As you might expect, all the milk substitutes cost more than cow's milk, and the powdered form is generally less expensive than the liquid. Many brands can be purchased by the case or in large tubs— buying in bulk almost always saves money.

Sovex Foods, Inc. has recently introduced a new product called **Instead of Yogurt**. This instant food is easy to prepare (just add water, stir and chill) and is a wonderful, non-dairy, gluten-free yogurt. It comes in five fruit flavors and will most likely make your yogurt lover happy. It does contain corn-based starch, so if your child has a corn allergy this product won't be tolerated. Although Instead of Yogurt has no calcium, it could be mixed with a (thinned) cup of a calcium fortified milk substitute rather than with water. The White Wave Company makes some delicious fruit flavored soy yogurts which are dairy and gluten-free. Look for these in the dairy section of your health food store, but note that unflavored variety does contain gluten.

When a recipe calls for butter or shortening, there are many options available. Fleishman's[2], for example, makes an *unsalted* margarine that is dairy-free (it is corn based, however, so don't use it if your child is allergic to corn). There are many non-dairy canola and safflower based margarines available, generally from health food stores. One excellent shortening choice is Spectrum Spread made by Spectrum Naturals. This spread is made from expeller pressed canola oil, and contains no trans fats (hydrogenated or partially hydrogenated.) It contains no dairy and has no cholesterol, but it does contain a small amount of soy. It tastes very good; you can bake with it but it will not melt, so you cannot fry or saute foods in it. These spreads usually contain soy lecithin so must be avoided by people who cannot tolerate soy products.

Sometimes, applesauce (or baby pears, if you are avoiding salicylates and arabinose) can be used in place of fat, but this will not always work, especially when making cakes and other delicate baked goods. There are also several prune-based products available that can sometimes be used in place of fat, but you will have to experiment to see if it works with a particular recipe. These are generally quite tasty and acceptable for the GF/CF diet. If dairy, fruits, corn *and* soy are being avoided, it becomes extremely difficult to find a fat that can be used in cooking and baking. One solution is to find cake and cookie recipes that use oil or mayonnaise in place of solid shortening; for cakes and quick breads this will be easier than for cookies, which generally require a solid fat. Try looking for recipes in Kosher cookbooks; because dairy and meat products cannot be eaten at the same meal, many desserts use oils so they may be served with either (foods that are neither dairy or meat are called *parve*—look for this word on products marked Kosher.)

Some parents of extremely food allergic or intolerant children have solved the shortening problem by rendering the fat from geese or chickens.[3] While this highly saturated fat may not be as healthful as other oils, it is sometimes the only choice when a fat source is needed (and all children need some fat in their diets). There is a big difference, however, between sauteing chicken in chicken fat, and using it to make cookies! Clearly the strong flavor of the fowl will be unpleasant in a cookie or cake.

Another choice is coconut oil, or coconut butter, as it is sometimes called. While we are accustomed to thinking of any saturated fat as unhealthy, *unprocessed* coconut oil is unlikely to raise cholesterol levels. Coconut oil is a medium chain fatty acid; because it is naturally saturated it does not have to be hydrogenated to solidify at room temperature. The process of hydrogenation creates trans fats. (33) Trans fats raise the bad cholesterol (LDL) and lower the good cholesterol (HDL) levels. Long chain fatty acids, which are stored as fat in the body, are associated with cholesterol problems. Further, approximately half the fatty acid of coconut oil is lauric acid. A component of human milk, lauric acid has anti-bacterial, anti-viral and anti-fungal properties. It is also a source of Medium Chain Triglycerides (MCTs) which allow the body to metabolize fat efficiently and convert it to energy rather than storing it as fat. For cooking or baking, replace butter or margarine with three-quarters the amount of coconut oil (see Appendix I for a source of unprocessed, organic coconut butter).

If a recipe calls for buttermilk, use the milk substitute of your choice and add a teaspoon of lemon juice to the liquid ingredients. In the past it has been very difficult to find a good substitute for cream cheese, sour cream or yogurt, but recently Tofutti Brand has come up with excellent non-dairy versions of each. These foods do contain both soy and corn, however, and cannot be used by people with multiple intolerances.

I am often asked if goat's milk, yogurt or cheese are acceptable for this diet. According to Dr. Karl Reichelt, the casein in goat (and sheep) milk is very similar to that of bovine milk and should be avoided. My own child is very sensitive to gluten but does not seem to react to casein. I try to keep milk products almost totally out of his diet, because of the similarity between the casein and gluten molecules, but (very) occasional use of goat's cheese and yogurt has not caused a perceptible reaction. According to Reichelt, if your child showed developmental problems from a very early age (infancy), you should avoid *all* milk or dairy products.

If foods, like countries, were afforded "most favored" status, cheese would certainly qualify. I can honestly say I have never met a child who did not like cheese and foods such as pizza and macaroni and cheese have been standards of childhood for generations. Unfortunately, it is very hard to find a good cheese substitute if you must avoid casein. There are many tofu, soy and even rice-based 'cheeses' on the market, but nearly all of them contain casein in one form or another. Soymage, made by Soyco®, is the only reasonable facsimile I have ever found that does not. It is quite rubbery, and does not actually taste much like cheese, but it does melt and can be made into a grilled sandwich or grated over pizza. Soymage can be found in blocks, or in individually wrapped slices.

Many people make mock cheeses with ingredients like agar or white beans (see recipes in Chapter 12). Sometimes, you can just fake it. I occasionally make 'macaroni and cheese' by covering rice macaroni with a GF/CF bechamel (white) sauce that I color with turmeric. For some reason I assumed, correctly, that since it looked right my children would not notice the omission. While it did not taste much like macaroni and cheese to me or Serge, it really wasn't bad...a testament that the power of suggestion can be very powerful indeed!

On to Gluten...

Removing gluten from the diet tends to be a bit trickier (and more labor intensive) than removing casein. Many of our children are addicted to wheat-based snacks—breads, muffins, pretzels, crackers, noodles, etc. For some of these, good substitutes are easy to find.

When there is no time (or energy) to bake, GF/CF breads are available at health food stores. The Food For Life® Almond-Rice, Pecan-Rice and Rice breads are quite good. They are generally available in the freezer case of health food stores. Ener-g® sells several types of gluten-free, dairy-free and even yeast-free breads. They are vacuum packed and can be found on the shelf or in the freezer of most natural food stores, and are also available through mail order. Although they make acceptable toast and bread crumbs, they are not, in my opinion, very tasty. If yeast is being avoided these breads are often the only available option. All of the commercially available breads are quite expensive—often over $3.00 or even $4.00 a loaf. (It makes the cost of a bread machine seem reasonable and many people who are serious about this dietary regimen do ultimately buy one—although it is not necessary.)

If yeast must be avoided but your child refuses to eat the commercially available loaves, try making sandwiches using quick breads. Be sure to cut back on the amount of sugar so they are more bread than cake-like. (Try the recipe for quick white bread in Chapter 8). I know of one mother who uses GF waffles for sandwiches, and her children love them.

If your child likes rice cakes, there are many ways to serve them and there are dozens of brands and flavors to choose from. Unfortunately, not all flavors of the brand most universally available (Quaker's) are reliably gluten-free. Call the company to check periodically, since production methods change from time to time. There are many brands available that are produced on equipment used only for GF products, so it does pay to call. There are also many rice crackers available that are crunchy and very good. Ka-Me brand is especially good and makes a great surface for peanut butter or other spreads.

Hol-Grain® makes plain rice crackers (ingredients: brown rice, water, salt) that are not quite as tasty, but when finely ground in a blender or food processor, they make excellent crumbs for breading or as a binder for burgers, meat loaf or stuffing. In addition, ground Hol-Grain® brown rice crackers make a great substitute for matzo meal. Two years ago I made delicious gluten-free "k'naydlach" (matzo balls) for Passover, and no one was the wiser.

There are many baking mixes available which make good waffles, pancakes or muffins. It is not hard to make these from scratch (see recipes in Chapter 8) but sometimes it is good to have a mix around. Fearn® brand brown rice mix makes very good waffles—a little cinnamon and a handful of blueberries or raisins added and they are a favorite with my children. Arrowhead Mills makes a very good mix with wild rice flour. Ener-g® also makes a good all-purpose mix (as do many of the mail order companies listed in Appendix I).

Many children react to apples, which are not allowed on the Feingold diet. If a urinary organic acids test showed excess levels of arabinose, you may also be avoiding apples. For any recipe that calls for apple, pear (which is lower in salicylates) may be substituted. If applesauce is called for, pearsauce may be substituted (see recipe in Chapter 12). Baby pears are also an acceptable substitute, but be sure to look for a brand of baby food that contains no added sugars, salt or starches.

When a recipe calls for powdered or confectioner's sugar, be sure to check the ingredients. Some brands use modified food starch and it is impossible to trace the source. Most specify cornstarch. If your child cannot tolerate corn, you can make your own powdered by grinding granulated sugar in a very powerful blender or a food processor. Be sure to grind in small batches, so you can get the sugar reduced to powder. If corn is a problem you will also want to make your own marshmallows, which is surprisingly easy to do (see recipe in Chapter 12). These make great eating, and can be added to cookies or other sweet recipes.

Frontier®️ flavorings are available at many health food stores and are excellent. They contain no alcohol, which most celiacs try to avoid if they cannot identify the grain it was distilled from. A few drops of Frontier maple flavoring into some vegetable glycerin makes a very good *faux* syrup for breakfast eaters avoiding both additives and sugar—this is even acceptable on a yeast-free diet.

Chocolate chips can be another source of problems. First, many contain milk. If your child must be dairy-free, you will need to find a non-dairy chip. Many use artificial ingredients, most notably vanillin. Vanillin is highly phenolic and should always be avoided (it is on the forbidden list for the Feingold diet too). In fact, it is possible that the problem chocolate poses to those with known PST deficiencies might actually be the result of using chocolate with this artificial flavoring added. There are several brands that contain neither ingredient (e.g. Tropical Source and Ghiardelli) but they do contain soy lecithin. If soy must be avoided, it may not be possible to find chips. If so, you can make your own by buying a high quality semi-sweet chocolate bar and chopping it into small pieces.

While most children can tolerate coconut and dried fruits, be aware that many brands contain sulfites. Sulfites have no function other than to preserve color and retard spoilage, and fruits dried without them are just as delicious. Read labels! Coconut will need to be purchased at the health food store—all major brands contain sulfites. Sulfites should be avoided whenever possible, especially if you suspect your child has a phenol sulfer transferase deficiency or asthma. Most raisins are not processed with sulfites, but some may be, so check your label. Also be aware that raisins packed in canisters often contain flour. Many companies dust down their equipment so the raisins will not stick together in the canister. Because the flour is not an ingredient in the raisins, it does not have to be listed on the label. If flour was used in processing, the raisins are most certainly contaminated—to be safe you should only buy raisins that are packed in boxes.

There are many excellent GF **pastas** available through mail order or in natural food stores. Pastas made from corn, quinoa and rice in various shapes and sizes can be found easily. These will serve as excellent substitutes for wheat noodles in all your recipes. Be creative with noodles! Did you know that you can make a delicious crust out of cooked spaghetti? Make corn or rice spaghetti, boiling only to the al dente state. Add two beaten eggs, mix it well, and place in a pie pan. Bake for a few minutes in a moderate oven, then fill with whatever you like—browned meat with marinara sauce is good—and bake again.

If you use breading to bind meat or for frying chicken, follow the recipe for Basic GF Breading in Chapter 7. It can be stored in an airtight container and used as needed, adding spices and other ingredients to suit particular recipes or your family's preferences.

Ethnic Foods

America is often called a "melting pot", and this cultural diversity is very beneficial to many of us searching for recipes that will fit our child's special dietary needs. An easy way to vary the diet is by borrowing from other ethnic cultures, especially those that are rice-based. Go to the library and check out cookbooks on Chinese, Japanese, Thai, Korean and Indian cuisine. You will find that many of the recipes will not even require modification!

Even familiar foods, such as rice, are prepared differently in distant parts of the world. Short grained rice (known as Arborio rice) is easy to find—italians use it to cook the wonderful dish *risotto*, which is delicious and different. It has a wonderful creamy texture that most children, even finicky ones, like. It can be varied in hundreds of ways, and whole cookbooks have been dedicated to its preparation. In many Mexican dishes, corn, rice and beans are combined in delicious recipes that contain high quality protein and no forbidden foods.

Asian, Indian and Hispanic grocery stores are wonderful sources of unusual or hard to find ingredients. In addition to carrying white rice flour and sweet rice flour, Asian markets also carry many types of rice noodles and rice wrappers. These wrappers are brittle, but when dipped in water for a few moments, become soft and pliable. They can then be filled with vegetables, meat or a combination of both, and made into little egg rolls or won tons. Indian stores often sell flakes rice (Pohu) which can be used much like oatmeal. Because it is crunchier than rolled oats, you may prefer to add it to a recipe's wet ingredients for a few minutes to soften. Flaked rice even makes mock oatmeal cookies possible!

Hispanic markets also have ingredients that can be used to vary and enliven the diet. **Plantain flour** makes a wonderful addition to breads, pancakes and waffles, giving them a subtle banana flavor. These markets also carry coconut milk, which can be used as a substitute for milk in some recipes. Many grocery stores also carry other items used in Spanish and Puerto Rican cuisine, especially if the neighborhood is ethnically mixed. If you can find such a store, look carefully at items that are unfamiliar to you. In addition to many rice, corn and bean products, you can also find unusual vegetables. My store carries fresh and frozen taro, malanga and cassava, all of which can be cooked and eaten like potatoes. Because these tubers (root vegetables) are fairly bland, they can serve as the basis of many interesting dishes. They are also suitable for a white diet, if you are trying to eliminate all (or nearly all) pigments.

Malanga is often considered to be the most hypoallergenic food in the world, because its starch grains are the smallest and most easily digested of all complex carbohydrates. Even children with extreme sensitivities should tolerate it. Malanga is closely related to the **taro** root, which is used to make poi in many Polynesian cultures. **Cassava** (also known as manioc) is a large brown root that is very white and fleshy on the inside. Tapioca, which most people are familiar with, is derived from this root. **Cassava must be cooked before eating—it is toxic when raw.** Flours made from these and other unusual foods can be obtained via mail order (see Appendix I.)

Many health food stores stock Rice Crust Pizzas, but most of these frozen pizzas contain casein. These stores also generally stock frozen rice crusts, which can be filled with your own acceptable toppings. Recipes for breads and pizzas can be found in Chapter 8. Several of the mail order companies listed in Appendix I make excellent pizza crust mixes. For a change of pace use corn tortillas and toppings to make Tostadas. These individual tortillas are delicious when topped with browned meat, beans, salsa and tomato. Many health food stores now carry pre-baked tostada shells, shaped like small bowls. My children get a big charge out of being allowed to eat their 'bowl' along with its contents.

If your child tolerates soy, you should learn about the many uses of tofu and the products made from it. Since the flavor of tofu is fairly innocuous, you can blend it and add it to sauces and casseroles—it will serve as a thickener, and will add a lot of protein. It even forms the basis for delicious, protein rich pudding or frozen pudding pops.

Baking from Scratch—Without Gluten

You've probably heard the old joke about the man who hurt his arm and asked, "But Doctor, will I be able to play the violin?" "Certainly, when your arm is healed." "That's great! I couldn't play it before!" goes the punch line. Well, if you cannot bake now, switching to GF and CF is not going to make it any easier!

But if you are already someone who bakes muffins, cakes or cookies for your family, it should not be hard to modify your own favorite recipes.

To do so, however, you have to understand what function gluten serves in baked goods. Gluten is an elastic protein. When you are making bread, the process of kneading the dough develops the gluten, creating stretchy strands. The gases given off by the metabolism of the yeast get trapped in the spaces created by this 'web' of dough, and push the dough up and out (in other words, the dough rises.)

In non-yeast breads and cookies, the dough is not kneaded; in fact, over mixing muffins or quick bread batter will begin to develop the gluten, which is undesirable. Developing the gluten in quick breads or muffins will result in holes and tunnels, and will make beautiful looking pancakes which are tough rather than tender. But even in these foods, the stretchiness of the gluten provides the necessary structure to prevent a cookie from disintegrating into crumbs the instant you pick it up.

Since the GF flours and flour combinations do not contain this protein, something else must serve the same function if the end result is to be acceptable. This is possible with the addition of **xanthan gum, methylcellulose** or **guar gum**. These ingredients can be hard to find—most health food stores carry at least one of them (typically xanthan gum). If you cannot find any of these at your local health food store, most of the mail order companies carry one or more of them. Guar gum has a laxative effect for some people, so xanthan gum is generally preferable. It is expensive, but because it is used sparingly, a little goes a long way. When converting a recipe to GF flour, add 1 to 1 1/2 teaspoons of xanthan gum for each cup of flour.

Many GF bakers also add 1-3 tsp. of egg replacement powder, powdered pectin or unflavored gelatin to their breads.

These ingredients improve the texture of breads. The texture of a baked product, often called the "mouth feel" is very important. Although you may not consciously notice the crumb structure and mouth feel when you eat a slice of bread or a piece of cake, these are factors which contribute to whether or not you enjoy the food. If you think back to some wonderful food you ate in the past, most likely you will recall the sensation of having it in your mouth—perhaps you remember that it was "silky" or "velvety." *If everyone notices these factors on some level, imagine how important such textural characteristics are for children (or adults) who have tactile defensiveness or other sensory disturbances.*

To achieve both pleasant tastes and textures in your quick breads, cookies, cakes, yeast breads and muffins, you will need to keep a variety of flours on hand. If you have never tried living without gluten, many of the flours will be unfamiliar to you. Some are native to the United States but used mainly for livestock or as fillers; others are borrowed from different cultures. For the most part, you will want to combine more than one type of flour when you bake without gluten.

Quinoa is a gluten-free flour that adds good body and flavor to baked goods; if used alone it tastes rather odd, so use it for no more than half the flour in a given recipe. (Some celiac groups contend that Quinoa is not gluten-free, but most agree that it is a safe food.) **Soy flour** is also good when used as part of a recipe's flour content, adding a slightly nutty taste and a bit of moistness, protein and fat. Since it tends to go rancid, buy it in small bags and store them in the refrigerator or freezer.

Brown and white rice flours are the basis of most gluten-free baking. Brown rice flour contains more nutrients since it is less refined, and it is sometimes easier to find, since many health food stores have a "no refined products" policy. For making cakes, breads and cookies, however, you need white rice flour. Arrowhead Mills makes one; since almost all health food stores (and many supermarkets) carry this brand, you should be able to get the store manager to order the white rice variety. Be warned, however, that this brand is not nearly as soft as some others (such as Ener-g®) and some children may not tolerate the somewhat grainy feel of foods made with this flour. Many stores carry bags of white rice flour made by Goya; this is a very soft, fine flour that will work well in GF baking. Asian markets are also good sources for soft white rice flour. **Sweet rice flour** makes an excellent thickener for gravies or cream sauces. Sometimes called "glutinous" flour, it does not contain any gluten.

In general, you cannot go wrong with Bette Hagman's Gluten-free Flour mix. This mix consists of 2 parts white rice flour, 2/3 part potato starch flour, 1/3 part tapioca starch. With a teaspoon of xanthan gum added per cup of flour mix, it can be used as a direct substitute for white flour in nearly any recipe. You should keep some of this mixture on hand at all times; it is easy to mix up a large canister yourself. If you prefer, Ener-g® sells it in one and five pound packages. It is available at many health food stores, or through mail order.

While Indians and Pakistanis might laugh at the idea that it is new, **Jowar flour** has recently been touted as an excellent gluten-free alternative. This flour is made from sorghum; many people say that, with xanthan gum added, it is interchangeable with wheat flour in most recipes. It is darker and heartier than rice flours—I would suggest using it in recipes that call for whole wheat flour. In general, I would recommend using jowar for only part of the flour in a given recipe; when used alone the end product tends to be quite heavy. American farmers grow sorghum, and there are a few American companies that sell it. It is usually available at Indo-Pak groceries, and is generally cheaper there.

Potato Starch Flour is available in health food stores and in the Kosher section of most supermarkets. Do not confuse Potato **starch** flour with Potato flour. The latter has a heavy flavor and the two cannot be used interchangeably in recipes. **Tapioca starch** is also widely available, and has a texture similar to **corn starch**. In fact, if your child is sensitive to corn, tapioca starch makes a good substitute. **Arrowroot** is a starch with similar properties, and I have yet to hear of a child who cannot tolerate it. This starch makes an excellent addition to waffle and pancake recipes—giving the finished product an excellent texture, soft inside yet crispy on the outside. Another alternative starch is **Kuzu Root Starch**, made from the wild Kuzu plant; it is rich in minerals and some people prefer it to arrowroot and other starches. Bean flours such as pea, lentil or chickpea combine well with rice flour, and are excellent additions to breading. Foods made with the more reamed flours (such as white rice) contain very little protein, but adding bean flour will significantly increase the protein content of your baked goods. They can also be added to meat for binding when making burgers or meatballs. Indian cuisine uses chickpea flour (called besan) to make a batter for dipping and frying vegetables (called Pakoras.) Lentil flour is the main ingredient for small Indian breads called Pappadam; these are crunchy and delicious. Pappadam mixes can be found at Indo-Pak groceries. They are also available pre-formed; to prepare them you need only fry in oil for a few minutes just before serving (they can also be baked). **Poi** flour (taro) is extremely digestible and is excellent if there are multiple allergies or gastrointestinal problems. It is a good source of Vitamin B-1 and calcium. It can be made into hot cereal or used as a thickener for soups or puddings.

Baking powder should be gluten-free. Some brands, such as Featherweight, are specified gluten-free, but others (e.g. Rumford) specify corn starch and are also acceptable if corn is tolerated.

If you have a favorite recipe that is usually made with wheat flour, you will probably be able to modify it for this diet. You will need to use one (or a combination) of the GF flours listed here, and you must add one teaspoon of xanthan gum (or one of the other gluten substitutes) for each cup of flour. Generally, you will also want to add structure by increasing the number of eggs in the recipe—if you want to avoid too much fat use only the egg whites for the additional egg(s), or use an egg replacer powder.

Often an increase in leavening is required when a recipe is modified for GF flours. An extra 1/2 tsp. of baking powder or baking soda may be sufficient, but to be sure you will need to experiment a bit. Another way to improve the results of baked goods using these flours is to make smaller loaves or cakes. You can divide a quick bread batter between two mini-loaf pans, or you could make rolls instead of a loaf. Larger baked products certainly can be made, but the smaller ones are often more like the real thing in texture.

Because different flours absorb different amounts of liquid, you may have to use more or less liquid in a recipe, depending on your choice of flour. The consistency of your dough or batter is what counts; try to achieve the consistency described in a recipe by adjusting the liquid. In general, use only part of the liquid called for, adding the full amount if needed. If the mixture is still too dry or too heavy, add more than the recipe called for, a few tablespoons at a time.

Make notes as you experiment so you will not forget just which modifications produced the best outcome. You may need to make more than one modification, and it may take a few trials, but in most cases you can duplicate your family's favorites fairly reliably.

Eggs serve many functions in cooking, but unfortunately, many children simply cannot tolerate them. While many egg substitutes exist, you must first determine the function egg serves for a particular recipe before you can decide which one is appropriate. For most recipes, Ener-g® * egg substitute will work well. This and similar products are made of potato starch, tapioca flour and baking powder, and are well tolerated by most people. If egg serves as a leavening agent, a teaspoon of baking powder for each egg in the recipe should work. In cakes, a teaspoon of vinegar can be used for each egg—this also serves as a leavening agent.

If egg is being used as a binder in muffins or quick breads, you can boil a tablespoon of flax seed or flax seed powder in a cup of water for 15 minutes, and add this as needed to your batter. Flax seeds can also be ground and added directly to baked goods—they add fiber and are an excellent source of essential fatty acids. Another way to replace eggs is to soften a teaspoon of gelatin in 3 tablespoons of boiling water. Stir until the gelatin is completely dissolved and freeze until it has thickened a bit. Beat until frothy; this equals one egg. Crumbled tofu works when cooked egg is required, if soy is tolerated.

Of course, nothing gives baked goods the structure and moistness of real egg—if you know the culprit to avoid is the egg yolk, egg whites are fine. For every egg needed, use two whites. If the egg white must be avoided, I would recommend using extra yolks only when real egg is really preferable (e.g. for cakes). The yolk is high in fat and cholesterol, so a substitution rather than doubling up on yolks would be advisable. If an egg allergy exists, be aware that an egg by any other name-well, you get the point! When you read labels watch out for ingredients such as: albumin, conalbumin, livetin, mucoid, ovomucoid, ovolbumin and vitellin—these product ingredients are all derived from egg.

Eating involves most of our senses, with input coming to many different sensory channels at the same time. The way in which our brain interprets these sensory experiences greatly influences how we feel about particular foods. To enjoy (or even try) a food, it must first be *visually* appealing to us. If we do not like the *smell* of a food, it is unlikely we will be willing to eat it. It has to *feel* right too; I have never liked pears as well as other fruits because they are too grainy and I dislike the sensation against my teeth and tongue. If a child finds a food too hard or too chewy, it may seem like too much trouble to eat. And of course, if we are to enjoy a food, it does have to *taste* good too.

It should not be all that surprising then, that some of these senses also give us important information as we are baking. If you are aware of your senses you will have more baking successes, whether you are using wheat or GF flours. For example, here is an old baker's trick you should be aware of— let yourself be led by your nose! Always open the oven and check for doneness when you *first* begin to smell your bread, cake, cookies or muffins. Good smells begin to emerge from your oven when the food is *almost* baked through; if you can smell it, it should be closely monitored from that point on. Most of us do not notice those first aromas; by the time we smell the food it is often a bit over baked, too dark or too dry.

Believe it or not, if you really pay attention to your sense of smell while you are baking, you can train yourself to start noticing those first aromas. After a while this comes naturally, and you will not need to concentrate on it. At first you may only notice the smell when the food is actually done (or overdone). Soon, however, you will start noticing those aromas sooner, when foods are not quite baked through. If the food looks done on the outside, but is still raw inside, cover the pan with sprayed foil and continue to test every five minutes.

Another sensory trick that works well with cakes, quick breads and muffins involves your hearing. *Listen* to your food! I know that sounds strange, but if a cake looks quite done and the toothpick test is equivocal (perhaps it tests very moist but not actually wet), hold the pan up to your ear and listen. A cake or quick bread that is still uncooked will have a steady, continuous crackling sound, that is rather loud when held close to the ear. A cake that is moist, but not wet inside will emit a much softer crackle. (A silent cake is probably going to be very very dry.) If listening to cakes sounds crazy, try this: the next time you bake a cake, take it out of the oven when you are sure it needs another 15 to 20 minutes of baking. Hold the cake up to your ear and listen for a few moments, then return it to the oven and bake until it tests done. When you remove the finished cake from the oven, listen to it again. From that point on you will be able to recognize the differences quite easily.

When it comes to bread, home baked recipes produce loaves far superior to anything that can be purchased. The recipes included in Chapter 8 will turn out good loaves, and you cannot miss with the recipes found in Bette Hagman's excellent Gluten-Free Gourmet books (note that most of her recipes are not dairy-free, but can be modified easily).

If you want to prepare freshly baked bread, but just cannot bring yourself to start from scratch, try some of the excellent mixes available from the mail order companies listed in Appendix I. Most of these mixes are easy to make (either by hand or in a bread machine) and the results are delicious. They are a good compromise between store bought and home made. Even if you like to bake from scratch, a few mixes are wonderful to have on hand for those days when you are simply too busy to bake from scratch. Many people on GF diets use only the mixes; they never liked baking and this is a good solution for them.

Other Things to Watch For

I cannot stress often enough that you must check all labels. Even if the food you are buying was OK a few months ago, ingredients and suppliers are constantly changing. Pringles® brand chips were once a big favorite for my son, but then wheat starch was added to the ingredient list and they have been off limits ever since. (Nearly all the low fat baked potato chips also contain wheat, which may be one reason that their taste and texture is so similar to Pringles®.)

Many prepared foods and sauces contain wheat, and other foods have gluten added. Anything containing **modified food starch** is suspect. Rice Syrup, a common sweetener, sometimes has extracts from barley. Canned soups often contain wheat, and of course cream soups cannot be eaten or used as an ingredient in casseroles.

Caramel coloring is questionable; if it is an American-made product, the caramel is probably acceptable. That may or may not be true for imported foods. **Hydrolyzed vegetable protein** is used in many products (labeled HVP). Sometimes it is derived from casein. Even canned tuna often contains casein derivatives! **Maltodextrin** is another ingredient that can come from many different sources. Often it is derived from corn, sometimes from wheat. I recently called a company to inquire about the source of the maltodextrin in a food and was told it comes from pine bark and chicory root!

Many people use Tofutti as a non-dairy ice cream, but be warned, it is not gluten-free. Rice Dream non-dairy frozen desserts are OK, but not those coated with carob or chocolate. Sorbet or fruit ices are better choices—there are many flavors available, including some from the premium ice cream brands.

Some **baking yeast** is grown on a wheat substrate—use Red Star or Saf brands when doing gluten-free baking. The Red Star yeast company will send you a booklet on baking without gluten; call 1-800-4 CELIAC and leave your name and address.

Be careful about contamination. Even a few crumbs can cause a reaction once your child has been GF for a period of time. In a restaurant, eggs could be contaminated with gluten from a griddle recently used to cook pancakes. At home, cross-contamination can also take place, when using the same utensils with safe and then unsafe foods (e.g. spreading jam on wheat toast and then using the same knife or jam for GF bread). Some people have two toasters, for gluten and GF breads. Others clean out crumbs after every toasting. Still others choose to buy or make only GF breads, so this cannot happen. A good compromise is a toaster oven—if you put all breads on a new sheet of aluminum foil before toasting, the chance for contamination is eliminated.

If testing shows that your child must follow a traditional anti-yeast regiment, further restrictions will apply. Sugar, thought to feed the yeast, will need to be greatly reduced (or even eliminated). This includes not only sucrose (table sugar), but also honey, molasses, fructose, etc. Yes—even fruit is limited on this diet. Most doctors will permit two, peelable fruits per day. In addition, anything that was fermented (e.g. soy sauce, tofu, tempeh and vinegar), fungus (mushrooms) or anything that grew on the gourd (legumes, melons, berries, etc.) are eliminated. So too are all gluten grains and baker's yeast. Carbohydrates are generally kept to a minimum. Fruit juices are strictly limited, and those that are allowed include small amounts of freshly made juice or unsweetened pineapple juice (juices from cans and concentrate generally ferment rather quickly).

Fortunately, most people do not need to stay on the yeast-free diet indefinitely. It is a particularly difficult diet for children to follow. Because of the restrictions on most forms of sweetening, most of the recipes in Chapters 10 and 11 are inappropriate for an anti-yeast diet. There are two sweeteners that can be used on yeast-free diets, however, in moderation. Neither is ideal for baking, but when a child is denied all sweets these will start to look pretty good, and they are worth experimentation.

One is **100% pure Vegetable Glycerin** (be sure to get 100% pure—lower grades are used in cosmetics but are not edible). This is a viscous liquid that will work best in recipes that use a liquid sweetener to begin with (honey, corn syrup, molasses). Another acceptable sweetener for this regimen is stevia powder. Stevia has been the subject of a bitter battle with the FDA, which has given it only limited approval. It has been used for many years in China and South America, but here the argument has revolved around whether it is a food or a food additive. Because no company can hold a patent on this natural sweetening source, no one is willing to spend the millions of dollars it costs to get a food approved by the FDA. Stevia has been available for some time as an ingredient in foods. It can be bought as a tea or as a dark, heavy powder or liquid, which has a definite taste and smell of anise. There is a white powder version available from a few sources (see Appendix I.) The sweetening extract (stevioside) is 300 times sweeter than sugar, while the herb itself *(Stevia rebaudiana)* is about 30 times sweeter. It has no calories. It is quite expensive, over $10.00 per ounce; but because of its extreme sweetness it is used in small amounts.

All of this may sound like a great deal to remember. It is. Once you know what to buy and how to prepare it, however, implementing this diet is reasonably easy. The hardest part may be eliminating all the shortcuts—the convenience foods on which busy people have come to depend. I have provided a few recipes for mixes which will help, and the mail order companies listed in Appendix I will be a big help too. If there is something you love to make, you can probably work out a shortcut for that recipe too.

But...Can We Ever Eat Out Again?

Yes, and no. Of course you can eat out but no, you cannot just open the menu and order whatever looks tasty for your child. It is obvious that crackers, breadsticks and rolls are forbidden, but you must be careful about other foods too. Many foods have hidden sources of gluten. For example, few restaurants make their own soup completely from scratch; they usually depend on a ready-made base that was purchased from a food supplier. These bases often have gluten in various flavorings, or other objectionable ingredients such as MSG, yeast or nitrites. Because the base was not made at the restaurant, the waiter will not be able to tell you whether or not the soup is GF, even if he knows what the cook added to the base. At many restaurants, they will not even admit to using these bases for their soups, so in general soup is not a safe choice.

Order carefully, remembering that the fresher and less processed the food, the more likely it is free of gluten and additives. Make sure that foods you order for your child are not breaded, or fried in oil with other foods that are breaded. Hot dogs are often on the children's menu—most hot dogs are not gluten-free. Check the labels on hot dogs available at your grocery store. There are probably ten to twenty brands available—of those, probably no more than two contain no wheat (or unidentified) starch. Further, hot dogs always contain nitrites, which need to be avoided. Many groceries and health food stores do carry nitrite-free hot dogs, but you will need to look in the freezer section. Since they are not preserved, they must be kept frozen.

We have always taken our children to diners—over the years we have gotten to know the owners of our favorite diner, and they make certain concessions to our needs. My son often orders eggs and fries, and when we know the people we can be sure that they clean off the grill first. I have even brought our own toast for Sam to eat with his meal. Another favorite item is the turkey plate special from the children's menu-we tell the waiter to hold the bread, stuffing and gravy, all of which have bread or wheat. Often they will offer extra potatoes or a vegetable to replace these items. You can also choose an appropriate item on the main menu and ask that it be served in a child's sized portion. Even though it may not be on the menu, most restaurant owners depend on repeat business, and will comply.

Like most children, Sam completely refused all vegetables (except corn, potato and tomatoes) for years. When he reached the age of eight, he decided he would give salad a try, and he loved it! Now, when there is little else he can eat, he is happy to order a large salad. Most restaurants offer their larger salads with grilled, skinless chicken, and that is a special favorite. Oil and vinegar are acceptable for a dressing. If and when your child agrees that lettuce is not an invention of the devil, try a small salad. (Do not forget to tell the waiter to "hold the croutons.")

We also eat at a local Chinese restaurant frequently. My son eats flat rice noodles (often called Chow Fun) with shrimp or chicken. We ask that they omit the soy sauce, since this condiment usually has wheat. We have wheat-free tamari (a form of soy sauce) at home, which is easily added to take out. He also enjoys the rice, so we order a simple stir fry of chicken and vegetables (again, *sans* soy sauce) for him.

Of course, if your child is like any other on the planet, the real issue is fast food. We all know it is not good for our kids, loaded with fat and sodium and low on nutrition. But tell that to a four-year old who has seen the golden arches! Generally, it is still possible to eat some fast food. The staff at McDonald's® and Burger King® are supposed to fry their fries In vats of oil that are completely separate from those used to fry (breaded) onion rings and McNuggets® or Chicken Tenders®. Be sure that they actually follow this company policy. Ask the manager if they combine the oils at night before straining and reusing. Do they use the same tongs to serve onion rings and fries? If the answer to any of these questions is "yes", do not buy the fries. One parent gave me the tip of asking for no-salt fries. These are always made separately, and you can always add salt yourself. Remember to call the companies too, do not just rely on the local employees for information.

Recently, the Burger King® chain has been test-marketing fries coated with milk and flour to improve heat retention and flavor. Obviously, such fries are definitely not OK for GF/CF diets! While the company did notify the major celiac groups around the country, no warning was ever posted for consumers at restaurants serving the new fries. Because consumers did not know of this test or where the new fries were being served, celiac groups and others referred to them as "stealth fries." Burger King received so many customer complaints (including those from celiac families) that the coating has been reformulated to exclude both gluten and milk. As of May 1997, the coated fries use rice flour and potato starch. The fries do contain some corn syrup, so if your child is allergic to corn these may still be off limits. As of this writing, the new fries have been introduced widely. The company is advertising their new fries, but if you have not seen any commercials touting them, be sure to ask at your local BK.

Breaded chicken is out, but most chains now have a grilled chicken sandwich. We order those without the bun, and though we are regarded as a little strange, we get it, packed in a little burger box w/tomato and lettuce. When we want chicken nuggets, I make them myself (see recipe in Chapter 8). My children both love them, and they can be frozen. If necessary, they could even be put in one of those little cardboard boxes obtained from your local fast food restaurant.

Sensory Disturbances

When you think about how important the senses are to the baking, cooking and enjoyment of your own food, it becomes easier to understand a finicky autistic child. These children are known to have great disturbances in various sensory channels. Some senses may be exquisitely sensitive; for some, touch is painful, and physical contact with other people may be avoided. If hearing is hyper-acute, sounds that do not bother others may be intolerably painful. Other senses may be far less acute than they should be. Great pressure on the joints may be calming rather than painful, and pressure or weighted vests can be used to provide relief.

For some children and adults with autism, such sensory disturbances are often at the root of their incredibly limited diet, preventing them from eating or enjoying more than a few foods. An overly sensitive tactile sense may make eating foods with varying textures or temperatures too difficult. An extremely sensitive olfactory system may make the ordinary smells of cooking (or eating) intolerable. They may simply not be able to get foods that you think smell delightful into their mouths. For others the opposite is true—the lack of a sense of smell may keep food from seeming appetizing. And although I have never read about this sensory problem anywhere, I believe that some autistics lack (or do not recognize) the sensation of hunger or satiety. I know of several autistic adults who eat by the clock, not because they feel the need to eat. These same people look at the plates of others to determine an appropriate amount of food to eat. My own son's Intake must be carefully monitored to prevent him from overeating. If he likes a food, he will eat it until it is gone or he has been told he must stop.

Of course, understanding how these difficulties contribute to the extremely limited diets of many autistic children does not really help to increase the number of foods that will be accepted. From the many parents I have met and spoken with, textural difficulties seem to be the hardest to overcome. In fact, a child may actually want to eat a particular food, but will gag or spit it out when the food is in his or her mouth. I have seen one child who kept reaching for banana; it was obviously extremely appealing to him. But he simply could not tolerate the food in his mouth, and spit it out immediately. Then he cried because he could not eat it!

If you believe such a sensitivity is affecting your child's ability to eat more foods, you should consult an occupational therapist who is familiar with sensory integration techniques.

There are oral stimulation programs that have been successful in gradually desensitizing the mouth. Therapists can gradually introduce new play materials with different textures (e.g. foam, finger paints, therapy putty etc.) so a child will also begin to accept new textures on their hands. Although sensory issues never prevented Sam from eating, he had many sensory problems including a very strong tactile defensiveness. Sensory integration therapy addressed this as well as other problems. Sam still has some motor difficulties and still uses a weighted vest to provide pressure, but he now tolerates all textures and is no longer insensitive to pain.

In addition to sensory integration therapy, there are several tricks that can be tried to increase the number of foods eaten. One is to introduce new foods with a texture and appearance very similar to another food already eaten. For example, if the child will eat chicken nuggets but no other animal protein, substitute a mild white fleshed fish, cut into the same size and shape, and dipped in a similar breading. Another trick is to introduce new foods that are eaten in a similar manner as the preferred foods (e.g. finger food, or soft food eaten with a spoon).

These are hard problems to solve, but help is available out there in the form of good therapy. I have also heard from many parents that after a few weeks on this diet (that is, when offending proteins or other food components have been removed) a child has begun to experiment with new foods on his own.[4] For some parents who have tried dietary intervention, this result has led to a much more nutritious diet for their child.

How to "Lighten Up"

Unfortunately, gluten-free diets tend to be rather high in fats. Of course children need some fat in their diet, and many kids who eat very few foods are quite thin. But the extra eggs, oils and margarines so universal in GF recipes are not in keeping with the dietary guidelines most of us try to follow. It is possible, however, to lighten this diet somewhat. Using various egg substitutes is a good place to start. Substituting ground turkey or chicken for ground beef is another way to cut excess fat—be sure that the ground chicken you buy was made of skinless white meat. If a recipe calls for browning the ground meat, you can cut down on both the mess and the fat by using your microwave. Line a plastic colander with 2-3 layers of heavy-duty paper toweling. Crumble the meat on top and place the colander in a glass pie pan or shallow bowl. Cook the meat until done, and most of the fat will have drained into the pie pan below. Place the meat on a paper towel-lined plate, and blot excess grease out with more toweling, taking care not to burn yourself.

When cooking chicken, remove any visible fat, and always remove the skin. You remove far more fat when you cook the fowl without the skin, rather than removing the skin after cooking. You can stretch casseroles, add nutrients and save money (by using less meat) by processing vegetables to a smooth puree and adding them to foods. Most kids will eat foods that have invisible vegetables added for flavor or as a filler.

In many recipes I suggest using refried beans since they melt into the dish when heated, adding flavor and protein without being obvious to children who are certain they do not like beans. Be careful, however, as many brands of refried beans contain lard. The cans marked vegetarian contain vegetable fat—look for cans labeled non-fat and read the ingredient list.

Dehydrated black and refried beans are available too; they are simple to reconstitute, have very little fat, and are very easy to use in casseroles and soups.

When a pan or dish needs to be oiled or greased, you can almost always use a vegetable spray instead (although for pancakes you will need to oil the griddle). If you saute onions or chicken, spray the pan and then add a little non-fat chicken broth to the pan rather than butter or margarine. If you are baking, use non-stick muffin tins, cookie sheets and cake pans. Whenever possible use parchment to line pans. Several mail order companies sell re-usable liners for baking pans, which are silicone coated and can be cut to specific sizes and shapes to match your pans. With lined and good non-stick pans, you should not need to actually grease a pan beyond a light spritz of vegetable spray. Often, the amount of fat can be cut in recipes for quick breads and muffins without compromising flavor or texture. If a recipe calls for 1/2 cup oil, try making it with 1/3 cup. Often, you will not even notice the difference.

By eliminating real cheese and milk, you have already removed two major fat sources in the typical American diet. Frying is another significant source, and it cannot be avoided if you are attempting to make certain foods (e.g. chicken nuggets). As long as fried foods are not a daily part of the diet, it shouldn't cause a problem. It may be necessary to go heavy on the fries and nuggets when first starting this diet, but once the child is actually eating, you should introduce new foods and cut back on the fried foods.

Most children eat far too much sugar—you can decrease the sugar in the diet by reducing the amount called for in most recipes. Some recipes will not work but many will be just fine. Try using 1/2 to 1/3 of the specified amount of sweetener. Once your children become accustomed to sweets that are not so sweet, they will not notice much differnece. Perhaps the easiest way to cut out huge amounts of sugar from a child's diet is to eliminate or greatly reduce juice intake. It amazes me how many children drink huge volumes of the high calorie, high sugar and nutritionally useless juices that fill whole aisles in most supermarkets.

If your child cannot give up juice, at the very least you should water it down. You can also make it yourself if you have a good quality juicer, adding in a few vegetables if possible. It is especially foolish to allow children whose nutritional cholces are limited, to fill up on these empty calories. The actual fruit is healthier, and in addition to the vitamins the whole fruit provides a lot of fiber. I often freeze freshly squeezed juices into ice pops, which are smaller than the usual serving and more fun to eat. If you feel you cannot remove juice from your child's diet entirely, make your own. If possible, stick to pear juice which is less phenolic than apple or 'red' juices, and water it down!

Foods You Can Eat on a GF/CF Diet

Fresh fruit (If on anti-yeast diet, eat only fruits that can be peeled, no more than 2/day)

Fresh vegetables

Dried fruit (without sulfites)

Coconut (without sulfites)

Potato chips (READ labels—some have wheat or starch)

Potato sticks (same as above)

Popcorn (not buttered)

Rice cakes (read ingredients, some are NOT GF)

Rice crackers (Ka Me, Hol Grain and others)

Fresh meat, poultry, fish, shellfish and game

Corn

Millet

Teff

Rice and rice products (pasta, bread, etc.)

Quinoa, noodles and flour

Amaranth

Potato (fresh, starch, flour)

Buckwheat flour and groats (Kasha)

Millet (pilaf and flour)

Soy (unless intolerant)

Corn flakes (if specified GF)

Yarns, sweet potatoes (and flours)

Sorghum flour (Jowar)

Corn meal (and polenta)

Most nuts (if not allergic)

Eggs (if not allergic or very PST deficient)

Beans

Lentils

Tapioca

Foods You Cannot Eat on a GF/CF Diet

Always Avoid

DAIRY PRODUCTS i.e.

Milk

Half and half

Cream Cheese

Sour Cream

Cream

Cottage Cheese

Yogurt

Hard and soft cheeses

Wheat

Bulgar

Durum

Spelt

Triticale

Oats, oat flour

Barley, barley flour

Rye

Semolina

Couscous

Wheat Pasta

Baking Powder (unless specified GF)

Soy sauce (unless specified GF)

Bouillon cubes or powder

Starch, Vegetable starch

Sauce mixes (read labels carefully, often contain wheat)

Malt, barley malt

Modified food starch

Rice Syrup (unless specified GF it contains barley enzymes)

Spices and herbs (buy only those specified free of wheat fillers)

Artificial colors

ITEMS MADE FROM WHEAT OR FLOUR

Bread

Crackers

Pasta

Pizza

Pretzels

Cake

Cookies

Chapter 6
With a Little Help From Your Friends...and Relatives!

If any dietary intervention is to be successful, it must be adhered to strictly. As explained in Chapter 1, it is only possible to determine if the diet will help your child, if all traces of forbidden foods and food components are completely avoided.

I know of several parents who maintain that the diet didn't help their children, but when questioned, it turned out that not one week of the trial went by without some infraction. If you "cheat" you will not know if this diet will help or not.

Even when parents are scrupulous about the diet at home, it only takes one skeptical relative, teacher, or therapist to scuttle the whole effort. And if this is done on the sly, you won't even know that the diet wasn't given a fair shot. Only when the diet has been kept strictly for a period of at least three months (Reichelt suggests a year) can you determine if the diet will benefit your child. If, after a fair trial, you see no (or very little) improvement, it is safe to assume that this intervention will not help. It is a hard diet to keep, and it would make sense to abandon it at this point, relegating diet to the "tried it" column that every parent keeps.

I do not believe that loving grandparents want to undermine parental efforts but many cannot get over the feeling that "Surely a little taste can't hurt!" For many grandparents, food = love, and the temptation is strong to indulge in giving some wonderful treat to a beautiful grandchild. This may be especially hard to resist, when the child is more receptive to such treats than to hugs and kisses. Perhaps the sharing of a sweet is one of the rare times the child actually *looks* into the eyes of Grandma or Grandpa.

Finding this understandable, however, is not the same as saying it is all right. In this case, a little bit **will** hurt! This means that you must work very hard to convey the importance of your parents and in-law's cooperation and support. The same problem may arise with teachers, therapists or sitters who believe they know a great deal about autism. They may never have heard of dietary intervention, or they may have questioned physicians and been told that special diets are useless. For these professionals in your child's life, it is good to have a written explanation of what you are trying to do. Though I wouldn't expect you to hand your mother a formal letter, the same ideas can be expressed informally.

Below is a sample letter—modify it to fit your needs and circumstances. I believe it would be appropriate for any professional who spends time with your child. Include with it a copy of the list of forbidden vs. safe foods which follows.

Sample Letter for Teachers, Therapists, Sitters etc.

Date:_____

Dear:_____ ,

I am very excited abut a special diet we are trying with (child's name- CN). Recent research in the U.S. and Europe has shown that certain foods may be affecting the developing brains of some children, causing or worsening autistic behavior.

Scientists believe that some autistic children have metabolic problems which prevent them from fully digesting certain commonly eaten proteins. This incomplete breakdown of proteins is very important, because some of them actually have 'opioid" activity. That is, they act like opioid drugs (e.g. like morphine) which affect brain functlon.

Two proteins in particular cause the most trouble. The first is gluten, which is found in wheat, rye, barley and oats, and any foods which contain even small amounts of these grains. The second protein is called casein, which is found in milk and all dairy products.

Since we cannot (yet) cure the metabolic error that causes this problem, the idea of the diet is to eliminate these proteins from the diet. We know that this diet won't   cure (CN's) autism but we are very hopeful that it will help with some of HIS/HER problems with (name some problems, such as toileting, tantrums aggression, remoteness etc.). I know that you also want to help (CN), and if this diet is to help we will need the cooperation of everyone who spends time with (CN).

It may seem as if (CN) will starve, since HE/SHE eats only ____, ____, and ____, and RARELY/NEVER eats fresh foods. But don't worry, I am learning to make acceptable substitutes for just about anything HE/SHE might ask for. There are also many suitable foods for sale at the health food store.

Because (CN) eats LUNCH/DINNER/SNACK in your HOME/THERAPY SESSION/CLASSROOM, I have included a complete list of what (CN) cannot have, and have made some suggestions for alternatives. I will be providing appropriate SNACKS/ MEALS for you to give HIM/HER.

The milk substitute I have chosen tastes good and is fortified with vitamin D and calcium—just like milk! Many other children who have followed this diet have realized great gains in the areas of self-help, relatedness, eye contact and in some cases, language. Although not all autistic children improve on this diet, many do, and I am really hoping that (CN) will too.

There is something we must all keep in mind as we begin to try this diet. Because these proteins act like drugs to many children, removing them may cause a worsening of behaviors at first, which is similar to the "withdrawal" that drug addicts go through. Some kids advance immediately, and some regress for a time and then improve. We will just have to try and see what happens.

I know that you will help us keep (CN) on this strict regimen. Though it seems hard, (CN) could truly benefit. If you would like to read some of the articles that I have on this topic don't hesitate to call. We're counting on your help, and as always appreciate your support!

Sincerely,

Your name

Copy the lists of foods your child can and cannot eat found at the end of Chapter 5. Append the lists to your letter.

Part II.
Let's Get Cooking!

Because my own son responded so well to a gluten and casein-free diet, I often feel exasperated when other parents are not willing to try it. However, I also know that I am lucky. Sam is not a fussy eater, and accepts the various substitutes I provide for him. He can now monitor his own diet to a certain extent, refusing regular bread or cookies. He also eats a wide variety of foods, much of it healthful. He takes the vitamin supplements I give him with little trouble.

So, where do you start if this does not exactly describe your child? If my child had an extremely limited diet, I would start with lab tests to determine whether or not he is likely to benefit from dietary changes (see Chapter 4.) These tests are not absolutely definitive, but positive results show that a dietary change may prevent further damage to the Central Nervous System (CNS). At the very least, positive tests indicate it is clearly worth the effort of at least trying this diet for several months.

All parents of children with limited diets want to broaden the food choices the child will accept; under any circumstances, getting a child to accept new food is a challenge. This challenge is *orders of magnitude greater* for many developmentally disabled children. It is frightening, when a child eats only three or four foods, even to imagine taking these away and replacing them with something unfamiliar. For parents of some special needs children, however, finding the courage to make these changes may affect the quality of their child's life for seventy years or more. When you think of it from this perspective, the potential benefits of the effort clearly outweigh the inconvenience and trouble (and tantrum!) involved.

When I removed the majority of my son's favorite foods from his diet, I did not know another soul who had tried this. It was over a year before I even found another parent with whom to share information (and recipes!). I kept thinking there *had* to be a book I could turn to, but even after extensive searching, I found nothing. Some of the books on Cellac disease helped, but of course our situation was very different. So, this book came to be...the book that would have been so useful to me four years ago. I wanted to provide other parents with enough information to help them decide whether or not to try a GF/CF diet. But, even the information alone isn't enough.

Nearly every week I heard from at least one parent who was anxious to try this diet—that is, until they went to the supermarket. Suddenly surrounded by all the foods they could no longer buy, panic set in. "What in the heck am I supposed to cook?" is a question I hear again and again. It soon became clear to me that advice on food, shopping, equipment and recipes was essential. This part of the book provides that information.

The recipes I offer should help you get started on the casein-free (CF), gluten-free (GF) lifestyle. Since so many children with autism are exceedingly picky eaters, it is almost certain that many of the recipes I offer will be, at first, rejected. Don't be discouraged, however. Many parents who have used this intervention with varying degrees of success report that its introduction was soon followed by a surprising broadening of the diet!

Some of these recipes (which no doubt *will* be accepted) do not win any prizes in the healthy food category. They are treats. Although I try, like all parents, to limit the junk food and sweets in my children's diet, this is very hard to do once they are no longer babies and you cannot control every morsel they consume. I do not feel guilty about this, because I believe that to have any hope for success you *must* be able to offer a treat. Most children will understand the concept of "No dessert until you have eaten 'X' bites of dinner." Furthermore, many autistic spectrum children are taught (at least some of the time) using applied behavioral analysis techniques described by Lovaas and others. For these kids. tiny bites of cookie are often used as primary reinforcers, especially at the start of learning, or when a task is particularly difficult for the child.

What if you are certain you can adapt your cooking, but equally certain your efforts will be met by a hunger strike? You may believe your child will starve. That *could* be true, but it probably is not. The important point to remember is this—since these children are so averse to trying new things, the trick is to make the new foods *seem* just like the same old fare. It takes some learning (and some mistakes along the way), but there is nothing difficult about preparing food that complies to the diet and is similar to the food your child eats now.

More variety (and less junk) would be a positive change in the diets most of our children are currently following. But if junk is what your child eats now, concentrate on making food he will eat now. Make a list of everything your child currently eats (unfortunately, that probably won't take more than a minute.)

Then, follow the guidelines outlined in the next six chapters to find ways to prepare acceptable substitutes. Use whatever trickery is necessary to make these foods seem like the food he or she currently eats (you will find a few pointers on this scattered through the recipes). Once you are certain that starvation is not imminent, *then* find time to work on broadening food choices.

I was taught, long ago, that "Cooking is an art, but baking is a science." and I believe it is true. After all, you can experiment with spices in a sauce or substitute vegetables you use in a casserole without destroying the essential character of the dish. You might not like the variation as well as the original, but it is a matter of taste and clearly not a failure. When you start baking GF however, failures are easy to define. Cakes fail to rise. Cookies fall apart when you try to remove them from the pan. Muffins are filled with holes and tunnels. Breads and biscuits are tough.

Experimentation has shown me that I can bake cakes and cookies as good as any I made with wheat flour and butter. This is important to my son—a child whose first multi-syllabic word was "delicious." And for poor eaters, you can always squeeze some protein or calcium into a dessert, which will certainly be gobbled up.

The recipes in this book will get you started, and should give you ideas about how to modify family favorites. Soon, such adaptations will come naturally. Once that happens, your own recipe files will become your best source of delicious, GF/CF meals for your family.

You may note that I have included no recipes for vegetables or fruits. Since these foods are fine for a GF/CF diet in their natural, unprocessed state, I would encourage you to serve them that way as often as possible. Most kids avoid vegetables anyway, but one day that will probably change. If they are available, organically grown produce is free of pesticides and ripening agents. Organic produce is expensive, so if you have the room and the time you might consider planting a garden. Even small towns often have food co-ops through organic farms—for a yearly fee you buy a share of the produce grown there. In larger cities there are weekly farmer's markets, where wonderful produce can be obtained. If you find organic produce to be prohibitively expensive, choose organic for fruits and vegetables that cannot be easily scrubbed or peeled.

When preparing produce, remember to follow the basic guidelines of the diet. If you typically steam vegetables with lemon and butter, use CF margarine instead. If you make a creamed style vegetable, substitute appropriate CF milk and thickeners for milk and flour. Fresh fruit is usually loved by kids, even finicky ones. Don't mess with success—if they will eat it plain, buy and serve it that way. If you are making a dessert with fruit thicken or bind with appropriate foods (e.g. tapioca or rice flour) and use special crusts and toppings.

Once you learn a few tricks, cooking and shopping will stop being such a chore. It won't be long until you are no longer bringing extensive lists to the grocery or health food store. This style of cooking will become second nature. Although it may not be necessary for your whole family to stay on this diet, try to make all meals eaten together comply with the diet. It is unfair to a child to see others eating foods he or she cannot. Don't buy wheat-based treats for your other children—not only is it cruel to your child, but they will certainly find a way to get to these 'forbidden fruits.' Your other children can get these treats at school or when they visit with friends. Explain to your other children how important this is, and ask them to help you with it.

If you are not already doing it, find a time *every day* when you can give your other children your full attention. You have no doubt sacrificed a great deal for your disabled child, but so have your other kids. Adding a restrictive diet may seem like just one more instance of their affected sibling's 'special' status in the family.

So, that's it! If you are ready to give this diet a try, read on for shopping and cooking ideas and general tips for making a smooth transition to a new diet. Happy cooking and eating!

Chapter 7
Dinnertime... Mains and Sides

Chicken "Nuggets"

No, they are not from you-know-where, but they are delicious. Your children should love them—these nuggets never last long around our house. If you feel you really need a deception ask for a few of the cardboard containers at your local McDonald's®. Since you can make as many or as few as you want, I give no measurements for this recipe. But my advice is make a lot! They freeze beautifully, and can be re-heated in the oven or microwave. I often heat these in the morning, and put them in a thermal jar for Sam's lunch. He insists they are still hot at lunch time, and they are a favorite.

Ingredients:

Boneless, skinless chicken breast

Egg (if tolerated)* beaten with 2 TBL. water

Basic GF Bread Crumb Mix (recipe follows)

Optional spices: Salt, pepper, garlic powder, onion powder etc.

Canola, coconut or other Vegetable Oil for frying

Slice chicken into strips, then into bite sized chunks.

Beat egg lightly with water and pour into a shallow pan or pie plate.

In another shallow dish, season Basic GF bread crumb mix with spices.

Dip chicken pieces first into egg, and then coat well in crumb mixture. If egg cannot be used, dip the chicken in melted CF margarine or in milk substitute. Roll each dipped piece in the breading, and coat well.

Fry in very hot oil, about 1/2" deep, until golden brown on all sides. Drain well on paper towel lined plates. Serve while warm. Extras that have been frozen reheat well.

Basic GF Breading:

Perky's brand Nutty Rice Cereal (finely ground in blender or food processor)

Hot-Grain rice crackers (finely ground in blender or food processor)

Mashed Potato Flakes (no sulfites, preferably organic)

Optional: Some people like to add chickpea flour to their breading. Blend ingredients in blender or food processor until fine.

Optional: GF Corn flakes, crushed but not to a powder

Experiment with the proportions of these ingredients until you find the breading mixture that you like. I generally use equal amounts of the first three, and add some corn flakes when I want more crunch.

For extra crunch and flavor, process roasted sunflower seeds—this is great when corn is not tolerated. Since sunflower seeds are oily and could go rancid, add these to the rest of the breading as you're preparing to cook your meal.

Make a large batch and store in an airtight container, since this breading will be used in many other recipes.

Fish Sticks

If your child will eat fish sticks, the directions are the same as for Chicken. Use a firm fleshed white fish such as flounder or halibut, and cut into rectangular sticks before dipping and frying.

French Fries

If you're going to serve chicken nuggets, you may as well go all the way and make the fries too. There are GF frozen french fries available, though you do have to read the ingredients carefully to make sure they have no wheat. Home-made fries are so special, though, they deserved to be made once in a while. I almost always make frozen fries, but in the summer when we have freshly dug potatoes from our garden, I like to make them from scratch. I slice the potatoes into the shape of chips (that is, following the shape of the potato) and that's fine with my kids. But if your child won't eat them unless they look right, you might want to invest in one of those gadgets that cuts perfectly shaped fries. Most kitchenware stores carry them, and they are inexpensive.

Ingredients:

Potatoes, peeled and sliced

Oil for frying

Salt

Slice potatoes into the shape and thickness desired, while your oil is heating. A deep fryer works best, but since I don't have one I always use a deep frying pan and about 1 1/2" of oil. I prefer coconut or canola oil—use whatever is best tolerated by your child.

Fry potatoes, flipping as they brown on one side, until they are brown and crispy on all sides. Place on paper-towel lined plate, draining the oil as much as possible. Salt and serve while hot.

Do not stand too close to the pan, and be sure little ones are not in the area—the moisture in the potatoes really makes the oil spatter.

If you want to, slice the potatoes as thinly as possible (use a mandolin if you have one). Fry as above. The result will be the best potato chips you've ever eaten!

NOTE: Kids need some fat in their diet, but if your child eats predominantly fatty foods, or if the whole family is to eat them, try baking the fries. Spray them with an oil spray, and salt them before they go into a hot (400 degree) oven. Bake until brown (timing will depend on the thickness of the fries, so watch carefully.) They aren't as delicious or as crispy, but they are very good.

Potato Salad

Fried chicken was always served with potato salad at my house. Not too many people I know indulge this way anymore, but once in a while...

Ingredients:

1 Lb.	Potatoes
2	Eggs, hard boiled and chopped
1	Onion, diced
2 TBL.	Drained, pickle relish (GF)
1 tsp.	Celery seed
2-3 TBL.	GF Mayonnaise
	Salt & pepper to taste

Place potatoes in a pot, cover with water and add 1/2 tsp. salt. Boil until soft but not mushy, 20- 40 minutes depending on size of potatoes. Cool and peel, then cut into bite sized chunks. Let them come to room temperature before adding other Ingredients.

Place potatoes in a bowl and add other ingredients. Use just enough mayonnaise to fully moisten. Chill before serving.

Baked Onion Rings

Onion rings lack the universal appeal of fries, but many kids will adore these. I am not sure Sam really knows what they are, but they are crispy and he thinks they are great. The adults at your table will think these onions are pretty great too. Since they are baked they are not too fatty or heavy. Use sweet onions such as Vidalias, when possible. Purple onions are also good.

Ingredients:

1-2	Egg whites or egg substitute
2 Cups	Basic GF Breading mix
1-3	Sweet Onions, depending on size and amount desired.
	Season the crumbs to taste

Slice onions into 1/4" rounds. Dip each in egg white and then dredge in the breading mixture. Place rings on a sprayed baking sheet, and spray the breaded onions too. Bake at 375 degrees for 12-15 minutes or until crispy and golden brown.

*For this recipe, add some crushed GF corn flakes to the breading if tolerated.

Salmon Burgers

When I was a child, my mother made these and called them salmon patties. We used to groan when she made them—it was never a favorite. But one night, when I was desperate for something to cook I found a can of salmon in my pantry and thought "Why not?" To my surprise, my kids and my husband loved them. I have to admit that they tasted a lot better than I remembered. Although kids do not usually love fish this may be an exception, and salmon adds calcium and essential fatty acids to the diet. Serve plain or in a GF bun or roll.

Ingredients:

14 oz.	Salmon, canned
1	Egg (or substitute), lightly beaten
1/2 Cup	Basic GF Breading mix
	Salt & pepper, seasonings of your choice
	Oil for frying

Drain salmon well and place in a bowl. Use a fork to break it up as much as possible. Either remove little bones or crush with your fingers—they are soft and edible, and add calcium. Then add the egg and seasonings. Mix well. Add enough breading mixture to keep the mixture together, and form as you would for burgers.

Heat about 1/4" oil in a 10" frying pan; you don't need a lot of oil. When oil is quite hot, place burgers in the pan, leaving enough space between them to turn easily. Fry on each side until well browned and forming a crispy outer surface.

Place on a paper towel lined plate and blot off excess oil. Keep warm and serve like burgers.

Salmon Puffs

These are a light and tasty way to get some protein and calcium into your child. They are so much like the previous recipe that I almost left it out. I decided to include both recipes, because some children may go for the fattier version and reject this recipe, which is baked. There is no reason you couldn't substitute crab or tuna for the salmon, and any of them would make a nice lunch or a light dinner. For a really smooth puff put the mixture in the food processor or blender until smooth, and then proceed.

Ingredients:

14 oz.	Salmon, canned
1/2 Cup	Basic GF breading mix (more if fish is pureed)
2 TBL.	Grated onion
1 TBL.	Lemon juice
	Pepper to taste
1	Egg
1/2 Cup	Milk substitute
1 1/2 tsp.	Baking powder
	Salt to taste*

Remove visible bones and skin from the salmon (optional). Add other ingredients and mix by hand or process until smooth. Form into small round balls and place on a sprayed cookie sheet. Bake for 25-30 minutes at 350 degrees or until brown. These puffs get very crispy on the outside, but remain soft inside.

*Because salmon tends to be salty, I never add salt to this recipe. If you want, add 1/2 to 1 tsp. of salt.

Crispy Baked Drumsticks

Not all kids enjoy picking up drumsticks—those with tactile defensiveness may find it unpleasant. But many kids do enjoy eating chicken with their fingers when Mom gives the OK. This version is low in fat, since it is not fried. You can also use this baking technique for nuggets if you want to. Simply cut skinned chicken breasts into bite sized chunks and proceed as for the drumsticks.

Ingredients:

1/2 Cup	Basic GF Breading mix (add crushed corn flakes if tolerated)
1 tsp.	Salt
1/2 tsp.	Paprika
3 lbs.	Chicken drumsticks
1	Egg, beaten with 1 TBL. water*

Heat the oven to 425 degrees.

Remove skin from drumsticks or breast meat.

Add spices to the breading mixture and place in a plate or pie pan. Put beaten egg in a second pie pan.

Dip drumsticks first in egg and then coat thoroughly with the breading. Arrange on a foil-lined, sprayed cookie sheet. Bake until done, about 45 minutes.

*If your child can't eat eggs, use 1/4 Cup melted CF margarine to dip chicken, or milk substitute.

"Mexican" Casserole

I am sure this recipe did not originate south of the border, but it is very good and a real winter favorite at our house. My mother uses it as an appetizer with chips, but I have always served it as a main course, with a salad and tortilla chips.

Ingredients:

1 lb.	Ground beef
1	Onion, chopped
15 oz.	GF Refried beans* (Dehydrated refried beans are excellent)
10 oz.	Salsa (check labels or make home-made-recipe in Chapter 12)
3-5 oz.	Mild green chilies, chopped
1 small can	Black olives, sliced
1 Tube	Cheddar style soymage cheese
	CF Sour cream substitute if soy is tolerated
	GF Tortilla chips, if corn is tolerated

Brown beef and onions, and drain well. Stir in olives.

In a two quart casserole, spread the refried beans to cover the bottom.

Over the beans, spoon half of the beef-onion mixture. Add half the salsa. Grate some soymage on top.

Place chilies over the cheese, and then cover with the other half of the meat. Cover the meat with the rest of the salsa.

Top with some more shredded cheese, then top with 4-5 TBL. CF sour cream substitute, if tolerated.

Bake at 350 degrees for 25-30 minutes, until the whole casserole is bubbling.

Serve with tortilla chips.

*Canned refried beans are widely available and come in non-fat versions (many brands have lard in them—besides being high in saturated fat, lard generally has a good amount of artificial preservatives). Check your health food store for dehydrated beans. They reconstitute with boiling water and taste very good. They also come in black beans, and these make an excellent casserole too.

Variation: Mexican Casserole with Chicken

An excellent variation of this recipe uses chopped, cooked chicken breast in place of ground beef. I use green salsa, which can generally be found at the grocery store (look in the Mexican food section). We often grow tomatillos (Mexican green tomatoes) in our garden and I make salsa verde (green) and freeze it. The plants are spindly and somewhat pathetic looking, but they are incredibly prolific. Four plants produce enough fruit to make salsa to last us through the winter, with spares for friends. If you cannot find green salsa, red would also be acceptable.

Tortilla Casserole

This recipe was originally a vegetarian dish, but since most kids won't touch something that is all vegetable, this version includes ground beef or turkey. You could also use leftover cooked chicken. If you prefer, you can use another (GF) grain in place of rice. When I make this all vegetable, I use refried beans to give body. We all like it a lot.

Ingredients:

1 Pkg.	Fresh corn tortillas*
1 Cup	Raw rice (white or brown) or other GF grain
15 oz.	Beans (canned), red kidney or the beans of your choice**
1/4 lb.	Ground beef or turkey

2 TBL.	Olive or other oil (only if making without meat)
1	Onion, chopped
1	Clove garlic, minced
1 Cup	Cooked corn (frozen or cut from the cob)
15 oz.	Salsa, homemade or a GF brand
	Grated cheddar style soymage
	Any other crispy vegetables your family likes

Cook the rice according to directions on the package. Set aside.

In a 10" saucepan, brown the meat, and then add onion, garlic and other vegetables except the corn; cook until soft. If you omit the meat, saute the vegetables in 1-2 TBL. olive oil (you can use fat-free broth if you want to omit oil). Add some salsa, to moisten. When mixture is cooked and quite hot, remove from heat and stir in beans, rice and corn.

Layer the bottom of a 2-quart, well oiled, casserole with tortillas to cover. Spoon approximately one third of the meat-vegetable mixture, and a few TBL. salsa. Grate some soymage or other CF cheese on top.

Cover with more tortillas, mixture, salsa and soymage for a second layer. Make as many layers as you like, making sure to divide the meat mixture evenly. Three layers is usually about right, ending with the meat and grated cheese on top.

Heat in a 350 degrees oven for 20-30 minutes until the dish is bubbly.

*My mother uses flour tortillas for this recipe, and it is delicious. Try the recipe in Chapter 8 for flour tortillas if you prefer, or if corn is not tolerated (and omit corn from the filling in that case).

** If your child won't eat beans, use refried beans. When you mix it with the vegetables (or vegetables and meat) it melts in and adds nutrition and flavor but isn't visible. You could also put cooked or canned beans into the blender or food processor to accomplish this, along with vegetables you want to disappear.

Easy, Low-Fat Tortilla Chips

It's easy to make your own chips for snacking or serving with these casseroles. These are lower in fat than regular chips, and have more flavor than the baked chips available in the store.

Ingredients:

1 Pkg.	Fresh Corn Tortillas (in the refrigerator section of your store)
1/4 Cup	Olive or other Oil*
	Salt, pepper, garlic powder, other spices of your choice

Stack tortillas and use a large, sharp knife to cut into 8 wedges.

Brush tops with oil. Place on baking sheet, oiled side up. Sprinkle with the seasoning of your choice, and bake at 400 degrees until lightly browned. They will be slightly soft, but will crisp up as they cool.

*To make a lower fat version, spray the tortillas with olive or vegetable spray rather than brushing with oil.

Shepherd's Pie

This is a dish my son adores. My version uses meat, but it can also be made into a vegetarian dish simply by replacing the meat with diced, sauteed vegetables or with cooked beans. If your child won't touch vegetables, you might cook some and puree them in a blender, and then add them to the dish. The nutrients are still there, and most kids will eat a vegetable if they can't actually see it.

Ingredients:

1 lb.	Ground beef (use ground turkey for less fat and fewer calories)
1	Onion, chopped
1 Cup	Stewed tomatoes, drained
1 TBL.	Parsley, minced
Dash	Worcestershire sauce (check ingredients)
1/4 tsp.	Pepper
4 Cups	Mashed potatoes, hot (instant, sulfite-free potatoes are fine)
1 TBL.	CF Margarine (optional)
	Grated soymage cheddar (optional)

Brown meat and onions, and then stir in all ingredients except for the potatoes. Mix well and heat through. Pour mixture into a 2-quart casserole. Grate some soymage cheese on top (optional).

Top mixture with the mashed potatoes, dot with margarine (optional). Put under the broiler for 8-10 minutes, until the top is just brown. Be careful that the dish isn't too close to the heating element, or it will burn very quickly.

Sloppy Joes

Most kids like Sloppy Joes. This is a dish I had completely forgotten about, until my husband revived it one night when he took charge of dinner. My kids prefer to eat it with a spoon, and eat their bun separately. The GF bun recipe in Chapter 8 works well with this dish, but any good GF bread is fine too. This just barely qualifies as a recipe, but Serge swears this is the best way to make it.

Ingredients:

1 lb.	Ground beef (turkey just doesn't cut it with this recipe!)
	GF Ketchup or homemade (see recipe in Chapter 12)
	Worcestershire sauce*
1	Onion, chopped
1	Clove garlic, minced
1 TBL.	Brown sugar, packed (optional)
	Salt & pepper

Brown the meat, garlic and onion, and drain off fat.

To the meat, add Ketchup, Worcestershire sauce, and brown sugar. Cook on low heat until the mixture is the right consistency, some sauce but not too wet, according to your preferences. Keep adding Ketchup and Worcestershire sauce to taste. Season with salt and pepper or whatever you like. Serve over GF bread or buns.

*Worcestershire sauce usually contains soy and/or corn products. 'Natural flavorings' may or may not be GF. Check with the company, and if a GF form cannot be found, you can substitute another flavorful sauce. Most sauces do contain some soy or corn however, such as wheat-free Tamari or Soy Sauce. Check with the various mail order companies to find a good GF substitute.

Spaghetti and Meatballs

Both my children love spaghetti and meatballs, but I was never a meatball maker or eater. My attempts fell short of the mark somehow, until my Internet friend Barbara Crooner shared her recipe with me. Make extra sauce to freeze and have on hand for other recipes.

Sauce Ingredients:

2	Large cans tomato puree (Contadina is GF)
2	Small cans tomato paste (unseasoned)
15 oz.	Can of tomato sauce
1 tsp.	Sugar
Seasoning to taste:	Pepper, oregano, bay leaf, thyme, parsley, basil and garlic are all traditional—use fresh herbs, chopped, when possible.

Mix all ingredients in a large pot or Dutch Oven. Simmer slowly and make meatballs.

Meatball Ingredients:

2 lbs.	Ground beef
2 1/2 tsp.	Salt
1	Egg
3	Slices GF/CF bread, soaked in water, squeezed and crumbled
3 TBL	Grated parmesan, if casein is tolerated

Lightly grease cookie sheet with olive oil (or use olive oil spray). Mix meat, and other ingredients with your hands. Shape into balls, and put on the cookie sheet. Bake at 375 for 10 minutes, flip over, and bake ten minutes more. Blot each meatball with paper towels, then add to the sauce. Simmer sauce and meatballs for 1 1/2 hours.

Pour sauce over cooked GF spaghetti (there are many types available at health food stores and through mail order) and serve.

HINT: If tomatoes are not tolerated, cook meatballs through and toss with plain GF spaghetti and some CF margarine. Season as desired. Many children prefer spaghetti this way, even if they can eat tomatoes. My younger son prefers spaghetti and meatballs served with brown gravy. ("Like they make it at school!") To make gravy without roast beef, use GF beef broth and substitute arrowroot or another starch for the white flour. Sweet rice flour also makes smooth gravy.

Simple Linguini

I made this vegetarian dish for a friend who had lived part of his childhood in Italy. He declared it was definitely authentic tasting. I don't know about that, but it is tasty, and few things could be easier if tomatoes are tolerated.

Ingredients:

1/2 lb.	GF Linguini (a good rice pasta works well)
1	GF Tomato paste, small can
2-3 TBL.	Olive oil
1-2	Cloves garlic, minced
1	Red pepper, chopped fine
1-2	Sprigs of fresh parsley

Cook the pasta, according to package directions, al dente. (If your family likes softer noodles, boil for a few minutes longer.)

Drain and rinse pasta then return to the pot. Toss with other ingredients in the warm pot.

Polenta Casserole

Polenta is a popular Italian dish, made of cooked cornmeal. Shortly after making polenta, it solidifies into the shape of whatever pan or bowl it was poured into. In Italy solid polenta is sliced into strips, fried in a little olive oil, then served with spaghetti sauce and grated parmesan. My mother saw a TV cook make a very complicated polenta dish and decided to make something that would be easier and faster to prepare. So she created this casserole, which makes a very nice change of pace from rice and other grains. Mom usually makes this as a vegetarian dish, but meat is a nice addition and a protein boost.

Ingredients:

1 Cup	Polenta (available in ethnic or rice section of supermarket)
2 Cups	Spaghetti sauce (GF brand or homemade)
2	Onions, chopped
1	Clove garlic, minced
2-3	Stalks celery, finely chopped
1	Parsnip, peeled and chopped
5-10	Mushrooms, peeled and chopped (omit for a yeast-free diet)
1/2 lb.	Browned ground meat (optional)
	Oil for saute

Prepare 1 Cup polenta according to directions on the package.

Pour the cooked polenta into a sprayed or oiled 10" x 13" baking pan (Pyrex works well, but you could also use a metal pan or a round casserole). NOTE: Polenta can be made ahead and refrigerated, as long as you pour it into the casserole while it is still hot.

Saute vegetables (use any crispy vegetables you like and have on hand) in a small amount of olive or other oil. Add browned meat if desired. Add spaghetti sauce and cook until bubbly.

Pour mixture over the polenta and serve. If the polenta was made ahead and refrigerated, place it in a warm (200) oven for 20-30 minutes prior to serving. If desired, grate a little cheddar style CF cheese on top and broil until melted.

Chili

*Chili made with meat (con carne) or without is another wintertime favorite at our house. When I was a child, it wasn't good unless it made your eyes water—I make a much milder version or my kids won't eat it. It was also made with ground beef but now I am more likely to use ground chicken or turkey, to reduce the fat. * Be sure the spices you buy are GF; you are best buying them from a company that guarantees this status. Many of the mail order catalogues offer GF spices.*

Ingredients:

1 lb.	Ground beef (or poultry or venison, if you can get it*)
1	Large onion, chopped
15 oz.	Cooked red kidney beans (or refried beans)
30 oz.	Canned tomatoes and juice, whole or stewed - check GF status
To taste	GF Chili Powder, salt, pepper

Brown the meat with the chopped onion. Drain meat and add other ingredients. The mixture will get soup-like after it cooks, but if you like it thinner you can add water or some thinned tomato sauce or salsa. Simmer slowly for at least one hour.

Be careful with the seasonings. Don't use too much at the start. After the soup has cooked for a time, taste and correct seasoning.

*Ground venison is very low in fat but has a much heartier flavor than chicken or turkey. It makes a great chili, but I wouldn't advise revealing the source of the meat. When a friend gave me some ground venison, my husband enjoyed it until he learned what it was. Some people just can't stomach eating Bambi.

Variation: Vegetarian Chili

Substitute cooked lentils or black beans, slightly mashed, for the meat. Cooked brown rice added at the end will add body to the soup, and completes the protein when combined with the beans.

Tamale Pie

Every chili lover knows that if there are any leftovers, Tamale Pie will make an appearance the next night! It 's a great way to use up chili, and tasty enough to make even if you don't have leftovers. Use whatever amount of chili you like, depending on how many people the dish must feed. You may have to stretch the chili with some salsa or other ingredients.

Ingredients:

Chili

GF Cornbread batter or Sweet Cornbread batter (see recipes in Chapter 8.)

Place chili in a one or 2-quart casserole, depending on the amount you have.

Spoon 1/2 recipe of cornbread batter on top, and bake according to cornbread directions.

It is generally best to use only half the cornbread recipe for this dish—if you have too much batter on top, the cornbread sucks up all the liquid from the chili. It's still good, but in this case, less is more. Use the other half of the cornbread batter to make muffins or a mini-loaf.

This recipe is good with either chili con carne or vegetarian chili.

Beef Stew

This is another of Barbara Crooker's recipes. It is very tasty, but of course some kids won't touch stew. You may be surprised however, and it is worth trying. My son loves anything with meat in it, and has even come to eat the vegetables (except carrots!) without making a fuss. Add any vegetables you like, frozen If fresh are not available.

Ingredients:

2 lbs.	Top round beef, cubed
1/3 cup	GF flour blend, or sweet rice flour
1 tsp	Salt
1 tsp.	Paprika
1/4 tsp.	Black pepper
1/4 Cup	Oil (to cut fat, use a non-stick pan with oil spray)
2 cups	Water
1	Small onion, peeled and chopped
6	Carrots, peeled and cut into small chunks

6	Very small onions (fresh or frozen pearl onions work well), peeled
6	Medium sized potatoes, cut into chunks
6	Beets, peeled and cut in half (when fresh beets are available)
1 Cup	Fresh green beans (when available), snapped and halved

Place flour, salt, paprika and pepper in a bag, and shake beef cubes in the mixture.

Heat shortening in a Dutch oven, add beef and brown.

Pour in water, onions and salt. Bring to a boil then reduce heat and simmer for two hours. Add other vegetables and cook 40 minutes more. If using frozen vegetables (e.g. peas or corn), add them just for the last five minutes.

Pizza

The Rice Council publishes many recipes and hints on cooking without wheat (using rice of course!). They have generously consented to my sharing a few of their ideas here. Most books on GF cooking include pizza crust recipes, and many of the mail order companies sell good mixes (see Appendix I). But if you want to whip up a crust from scratch, this is a good and easy one.

Crust Ingredients:

2 1/2 Cups	Rice flour
1/4 oz.	GF quick rise yeast (Red Star or Saf brands)
1 tsp.	Salt
1 tsp.	Xanthan gum
1 1/4 Cup	Warm water

1 TBL.	Honey
3 TBL.	Olive oil (use a different oil if it's better tolerated.)
1 Cup	Spaghetti sauce (GF or homemade) Cornmeal (if tolerated)

Combine flour, yeast, salt and xanthan gum in a large bowl. Stir in 1 cup of the water, olive oil and honey. Work the dough with your hands (it will be soft and crumbly). Add just enough of the remaining 1/4 cup of water to hold the mixture together.

Knead the dough in a bowl for five minutes. Cover, and let the dough rest for ten minutes.

Lightly grease a 12" pizza pan and sprinkle with a small handful of cornmeal. Flatten dough into a round disk and then press dough into pan.

Topping the Pizza

Toppings are limited only by your imagination, or what your child likes and tolerates.

Before adding other toppings, slice some mozzarella-style soymage and place directly on the crust. Add sauce and any other toppings you like, e.g.:

Sliced tomatoes	Slice onions (sauteed till soft)
Ground beef, browned	Sliced zucchini
Sliced peppers (yellow or red)	
Herbs, salt, pepper	

Grate some more cheese on top, and bake in a 425 oven for 25-30 minutes or until the crust is golden and the cheese is melted. Timing will vary according to the number and amount of toppings. Use a sharp knife or pizza wheel to slice into wedges.

Yeast-Free Pizza Crust I

*Beth Crowell is the mother of autistic triplets! She has worked tirelessly to find ways to help them (and other children) and soon realized they had severe metabolic problems. With a degree and experience in biochemistry, Beth was well suited to researching this topic. But that's not all—she and her husband are both graduates of the renowned Culinary Institute of America (the **other** CIA!). Together they published a book called **Dietary Intervention as a Therapy in the Treatment of Autism and Related Developmental Disorders.*** It is filled with much information on the research she has done and has many great recipes. Beth has allowed me to use a few of her recipes here; the one that follows is a real favorite. It is easy quick to make, and delicious. I always make the mini-crust version and my son loves them. If there are any extras, we eat them instead of bread.*

Ingredients:

2 Cups	Water
1/4 Cup	Olive oil
1 1/2 tsp.	Cider or Rice Vinegar
2 TBL.	Sugar
2 tsp.	Baking powder
2 tsp.	Garlic Salt
2 tsp.	Xanthan gum
2 Cups	Beechnut® Baby Rice cereal
2 Cups	Rice flour

Combine the first three ingredients in a large bowl. Set aside.

Combine the remaining ingredients, and add them to the oil mixture. Mix until thoroughly combined.

Divide batter evenly between two sprayed pizza pans and bake at 400 for 10-15 minutes. Remove from the oven, add sauce and top as desired. Return to the oven and bake until light brown around the edges.

For mini-pizzas:

Using 1/4 to 1/2 cup batter per crust, spoon onto a sprayed cookie sheet. Cut out squares of wax paper, spray them and put the sprayed side on the dough. Use a 6" sauce pan to flatten them, then remove the paper. (You can use the back of a wet spoon if you prefer.) Bake as for large crusts.

After baking, but before topping, the crusts may be cooled and frozen for later use.

*To order this book, send $14.95 plus 2.00 S & H to: Beth Crowell, 208 South Street - PO Box 801, Housatonic, MA 01236-0801.

Yeast-Free Pizza Crust II

This is another pizza crust with no yeast. It 's quite different from Beth 's crust, and is quite tasty if made very thin. It also has the benefit of being quick to prepare, since it has only a few ingredients and no yeast to rise. I once made this crust and forgot to add the baking powder. Amazingly, it seemed fine to me...perhaps a little flat, but every bit was eaten.

Ingredients:

1 Cup	Chickpea flour or other bean flour (see Appendix I)
1/2 Cup	Sweet Rice flour or baby rice cereal (no fillers or sugar added)

2 TBL.	Vegetable oil
2 tsp.	Baking powder
1/2 tsp.	Garlic powder
1/2 Cup	Water
To taste	Salt

In a large bowl, sift flours, seasonings and baking powder.

Make a well in the center and pour oil and water into it. Mix thoroughly and spread into a large round on a greased cookie sheet (wet hands to prevent sticking).

Prior to baking, add toppings of your choice. Bake in a 450 oven until the crust begins to brown, approximately 15-20 minutes, and toppings are cooked. You can also form this into four mini-pizzas. For children, I usually top only with grated cheddar and mozzarella style soymage.

Mock Mac & Cheese

I have never met a child who doesn't like macaroni and cheese. Unfortunately, both the wheat macaroni and the cheese sauce are forbidden on this diet. Soymage makes a decent substitute. The white sauce (bechamel) can be used as a base for any creamed casserole or soup.

Ingredients:

1/2 lb.	GF Macaroni
1	Onion, chopped fine
1/2	Package cheddar style soymage cheese, grated (optional)
2-3	Dashes of GF Worcestershire sauce (optional)
1 TBL.	CF margarine (optional)

Salt & pepper to taste

1 Cup   White sauce (recipe follows)

Make the White Sauce:

Melt 2 TBL. CF margarine in a small sauce pan.

Add 2 TLB. Sweet rice flour and blend into a paste.

Add 1 Cup milk substitute* very gradually, stirring constantly.

Continue stirring, and cook over medium heat until the sauce is smooth and thickened.

Add 1/2 tsp. of salt (or to taste).

*A thicker milk, such as soy or potato milk is preferable to rice milk for this recipe.

Finish the Casserole:

Cook macaroni al dente according to package directions. Drain, rinse and drain again.

Place cooked noodles in a small, ovenproof casserole.

Stir in chopped onion, Worcestershire (omit if you can't find a GF Worcestershire), white sauce, salt and pepper. Mix well and dot with the CF margarine, if desired.

Bake in a 350 degrees oven until warmed through, 20-30 minutes.

If desired, top with crumbled potato chips, extra grated soymage or GF breading mixture (into which a little melted CF margarine has been added).

Variation: Soy-Free Moc Mac & Cheese

Make as directed above, but leave out the soymage.

Stir 1-2 TBL. turmeric into the white sauce. This will give the sauce the color of macaroni and cheese, without changing the flavor too much. If you use no cheese product at all, you will need to add a little more salt and perhaps other spices.

You can also use one of the cheese recipes given in Chapter 12.

Arroz con Pollo

My friend Harriet Barnett has been cooking GF and CF for her son Andrew for several years. I 'met' her several years ago when I read a letter she'd written to Bernard Rimland's ARRI newsletter, looking for others following this regimen. I wrote to her and soon we were phone pals, speaking periodically. Later we switched to email and more regular communication, and last year I had the pleasure of actually meeting Harriet and her daughter Lauren. She has shared many recipes with me, and here is one of Andrew's favorites.

Ingredients:

1 lb.	Chicken (I prefer to use boned, skinless breast meat)
3 TBL	Olive oil
1	Red pepper, chopped fine
1 1/2 Cups	Rice (raw)
1 tsp.	Garlic (freshly minced, or use powder or bottled)
2 tsp.	Paprika
1 TBL.	Parsley, minced or dried
3 Cups	Chicken stock (homemade of GF canned)
1 1/2 Cups	Canned tomatoes with juice

Heat olive oil and saute the chicken. Add red pepper and rice, stirring to coat.

Add remaining ingredients and stir. Bring to a boil, then lower heat, cover and simmer for 25-30 minutes.

Baked Rice

Another of Andrew Barnett's favorites, here is one more way to cook and enjoy rice. Jacob will not eat anything green, so I put my fresh herbs in a tiny cotton bag that imparts the flavor without 'contaminating' it! The French call such a bag a "bouquet garni," and you can use this method for any recipe that calls for fresh herbs or spices you do not want people to eat, e.g. whole cloves, dried chili peppers. Look in kitchenware stores for the little bags or fashion your own with cheesecloth. NOTE: This recipe starts on top of the stove and finishes in the oven.

Ingredients:

2 TBL.	Oil
1	Onion, minced
1 Cup	Arborio rice (available in most groceries and in gourmet shops)
1 1/4 Cups	Clam juice or Chicken stock
1 Cup	Water
2 TBL.	Parsley

Preheat oven to 400.

Heat oil in an ovenproof saucepan, and add onion. (You can also saute some garlic if you like.)

Cook over high heat for about two minutes, or until onion is soft, stirring. Add rice and stir to coat. Add liquid, parsley and a large pinch of salt.

Bring to a boil, stirring. Cover and bake in the oven for 20 minutes.

Risotto

Long a favorite in Italian homes, risotto is finding a spot in American kitchens at last. A delicious, creamy form of white rice, risotto can be made with almost any ingredient added. There are even cookbooks devoted entirely to variations of the basic dish. It is a little labor intensive, since it requires constant attention while it cooks. I think you will find it well worth the effort. Make the rice after the table is set and all other food is ready to serve, so it can be put on the table as soon as it is finished.

Ingredients:

4 3/4 Cups	Vegetable or Chicken stock
1/2 Cup	Japanese rice wine (the alcohol cooks out)
1/2 lb.	Arborio rice
1	Onion, chopped
1	Clove garlic, minced
1 1/2 TBL.	Olive oil
1 tsp.	Salt
1/2 tsp.	Pepper
1 TBL.	Fresh basil, chopped *or*
1/2 TBL.	Dried basil

Optional: sliced mushrooms (not for yeast-free diet), finely chopped peppers, pitted, sliced black olives; 1 3/4 cup corn kernels (thawed or freshly cut from the cob.)

Combine the stock and wine in a saucepan, heat to simmer.

Saute rice, onion and garlic in oil until rice just starts to brown and the onion is soft.

Begin adding stock, 1/2 cup at a time. With each addition of liquid, cook while stirring, until the liquid is absorbed. Then add another 1/2 cup of liquid and continue this process until you have used most of the liquid, and the rice is creamy and soft.

Add seasonings and any optional ingredients. Continue to stir until the whole dish is heated through. Adjust seasonings and serve.

Kasha Pilaf

Kasha is made from Buckwheat groats and is available in the Kosher section of most supermarkets. Some argue that it might have gluten, but it is not closely related to wheat, and has never caused a reaction in my son. Buckwheat flour is sometimes produced in factories that also package wheat flours, and contamination has probably led to the idea that buckwheat products are not safe. However, most companies that make Kasha make little else and contamination isn't a problem. Call the company if you are unsure. Kasha has a nutty flavor and makes a wonderful different grain to serve alone, or as an ingredient in other recipes.

Ingredients:

2 TBL.	CF margarine
1/2 Cup	Chopped onion
1/2 tsp.	Minced garlic
1 Cup	Kasha
1/2 tsp.	Thyme
2	Sprigs fresh Parsley
1 3/4 Cups	Chicken or vegetable broth
1	Bay leaf
	Salt, pepper

Heat 1 TBL. Margarine; add the onions and garlic. Cook until the onion is wilted and soft.

Add the Kasha and seasonings, and stir to coat all the grains.

Add the broth and bring to a boil. Lower heat and cover, simmering 10 minutes or until broth is absorbed and the grains are plump. Remove parsley sprigs and bay leaf.

Add the remaining tablespoon of margarine and some minced parsley if desired.

NOTE: making plain kasha follows the same procedure with two important differences. First, prior to frying the raw grain, a beaten egg is stirred into it. The egg-coated grain is then heated until each grain is separate. At that point, add boiling broth (2 Cups water for 1 Cup Kasha) and stand back, it will spatter! Cover and simmer as above.

The other difference is that onions are the only vegetable added, and salt the only seasoning. Kasha can be used in most recipes that call for cooked rice. Add some small cooked noodles and you have Kasha Vamishkes. It is an excellent complement to roast beef—my favorite way to serve it is to cut the meat into bite sized chunks and mix it with cooked Kasha and gravy made from the juice of the roast (use sweet rice flour instead of wheat flour for gravy). Mix in any vegetables you cooked with the beef.

Riz Cous

When we still ate wheat, couscous was one of my son's very favorite foods. It cooks quickly and is very tasty, and we ate it far more often than rice. I was thrilled when Lundenberg Family Farms began selling Riz Cous, a rice based version, and devastated when it disappeared from my grocery shelves. Electronic mail to the company revealed that the product had been discontinued! All was not lost though, since Ms. Karen

Skupowski, a Lundberg employee, told me how to make Riz Cous for myself. It is fairly easy to do and worth a little trouble. You can make a lot of the dry Riz Cous, storing it in an airtight container, to be cooked and used as needed.

This really isn't a recipe, but rather a procedure to be followed. **The only ingredient is raw brown rice.**

Grind desired amount of rice in a blender or food processor. The resulting rice should look like tiny pebbles—do not reduce to a powder.

Place ground rice on a flat baking sheet, and roast at 350 for about 30 minutes. You want it to brown but not burn, and you will need to keep a close watch and stir it several times. This process releases the oils in the rice and is absolutely necessary for making a product that is similar to couscous.

Cool and store roasted rice in an airtight jar or other container. It does not need refrigeration.

To Cook Riz Cous:

Ingredients:

1 1/2 Cups	Water
3/4 Cup	Riz cous
1/2 tsp.	Salt
1 TBL.	CF margarine *or* Olive oil

Combine all ingredients in a saucepan. Stirring occasionally, bring to a boil and immediately reduce heat to a simmer.

Simmer just until liquid is barely absorbed. Reduce heat to low, cover and cook for five minutes. Remove from heat and fluff with a fork. Leave uncovered for five minutes, turn into serving dish and fluff again.

Chapter 8
Breads and Breakfasts

For many people just beginning to cook gluten-free, breakfast seems to be the easiest meal to manage. The following recipes for quick breads, muffins, pancakes, biscuits and rolls should help get you started. Most pancake batter will work well for waffles, so try that if your children prefer them. Muffin Top pans can be found wherever muffin tins are sold, and make only the rounded top. They have the added advantage of making small muffins, which look a little bit like fat cookies. If you use these pans, you will need to decrease baking time a little, since the volume of batter is smaller. When baking muffins, fill the muffin cups of your pan as directed. Any empty cups should be filled with 1/4 to 1/2 cup of water. This will help the muffins stay moist and prevents the pan from warping.

I have included only a few yeast bread recipes, since so many people avoid yeast. For a huge assortment of wonderful gluten-free yeast breads, I recommend *The Gluten-Free Gourmet* and *More From the Gluten-Free Gourmet* by Bette Hagman, published by Holt and widely available. I have also included a few recipes for unusual items.

If a recipe calls for GF Flour it means that I make it with the Hagman GF flour mix. If you prefer, you can use other flours or combinations of flours, but remember, different kinds of flours absorb different volumes of liquid. Try to get the consistency as described in the recipe, which may mean using a little more or less water or milk. It is often advisable to use a little less than the full amount of liquid, adding more as needed to achieve the proper consistency of the batter or dough.

Milk substitute refers to liquid; when powdered milk substitute is required, the recipe will specify *dry milk substitute*. For recipes calling for maple syrup, be sure to use pure syrup, not the corn syrup and flavoring concoctions sold under the big brand names. Or make mock syrup by adding a few drops of a strong GF maple flavoring to 100% Pure Vegetable Glycerin. (This can be used to lightly sweeten foods for a yeast-free diet.)

Some celiac groups advise against using vanilla and other extracts because they contain grain alcohol, which might be a source of gluten. I am convinced that these are not a problem. The amount Is minuscule, if it exists at all (some experts believe that the distilling process eliminates the protein from alcohol used in extracts). To be absolutely safe you may want to look for a good line of alcohol-free flavorings, such as those made by Frontier®. When I first began to bake gluten-free, I only used these flavorings. Later, I began to use vanilla extract again and have never noted a reaction. Do not, however, use imitation vanilla or any other food that contains vanillin.

Be sure to review Chapter 5 for general tips on baking with gluten and casein-free ingredients.

Karyn's Pancakes

Karyn Seroussi created these pancakes, and points out that they make excellent crepes. To make crepes, decrease the flour to 1 cup.

Ingredients:

2   Eggs

3/4 Cup	Dry milk substitute (DariFree is recommended)
1 TBL.	Oil
1/4 tsp.	Salt
1/2 Cup	Arrowroot powder
1/4 cup	Sugar
1 1/2 Cups	GF Flour (buckwheat is particularly good)
1 tsp.	GF Baking powder

Blend all ingredients except baking powder. Add baking powder and stir just a few seconds to incorporate it into the batter.

Spoon on to a hot, oiled griddle and cook until bubbles form. Flip and cook on second side and serve with syrup or fruit.

Don Baker's Pancakes

Don Baker has been making pancakes since he was seven years old. He can remember making chocolate ones for his little brother back then. I don't want to give away his age, but let's just say he's been making pancakes for a long time! When Don's wife Mary wanted to try a GF/CF diet for their son Alan, Don adjusted his recipe and the whole family continues to eat them. They are tender and delicious, with just a little sweetness added. My son likes to grab a few and eat them plain, as a snack. A few teaspoons of 100% pure vegetable glycerin would make this acceptable for a yeast-free diet. Extras freeze nicely.

Ingredients:

Dry Mixture:

| 3 Cup | GF flour mix |
| 2 tsp. | Xanthan gum |

1/2 tsp.	Salt
1 TBL.	Baking powder
3 TBL.	Sugar

Wet Mixture:

3	Eggs
1 1/4 Cups	(or more) Milk substitute
3 TBL.	Oil or melted CF margarine
1/4 tsp.	Vanilla

Combine dry Ingredients in a large bowl. Stir well.

Combine liquid ingredients in a bowl and mix well. Add to dry mixture and stir until there are no bumps, but do not over mix. The batter should not be runny, but should plop from the spoon. If necessary, add more milk, a little at a time, to reach this consistency.

Heat an oiled frying pan and drop batter in. Smaller pancakes are easier to turn, but if you prefer you can make large ones. Cook thoroughly until bubbles form and then flip to cook the second side. Serve with fruit or maple syrup.

Banana (Nut) Pancakes

This is a recipe from the U.S. Rice Council. The nuts can be omitted if your family doesn't tolerate (or like) them. Because the only sweetener is honey, you could easily turn this into a recipe for a yeast-free diet by substituting 100% Pure Vegetable Glycerin. Whenever I have a banana that's past its prime I peel it, cover with plastic wrap and toss it in the freezer. This way I always have it on hand, ready to use for banana bread, muffins or pancakes. They thaw in a few minutes and mash easily. You can also use babyhood bananas, but find a brand that doesn't add starch or sugars.

Ingredients:

1 1/2 Cups	Rice flour
2 tsp.	Baking powder
1 tsp.	Salt
1/2 tsp.	Xanthan gum
1 1/4 Cups	Water
3 TBL.	Vegetable oil
2 TBL.	Honey
2	Egg yolks, beaten
2 (large)	Bananas, mashed (or one 6 oz. jar baby bananas)
1/2 Cup	Chopped walnuts (optional)
2	Egg whites

Combine dry ingredients in a medium bowl. Stir in water, oil, honey, egg yolks, bananas and nuts.

Beat egg whites in another bowl, until stiff peaks form. Fold egg whites into batter and bake pancakes in a hot, oiled griddle or frying pan. Cook on both sides until golden.

HINT: Separating the eggs and beating the whites as directed, makes a lovely light pancake. But if you're in a hurry, this step isn't necessary. I often throw this batter together without beating the whites separately, and the result is delicious and tender pancakes that my boys love.

Gluten-Free/Rice-Free Muffins

If your child is on a rotation diet, you need to be able to make some foods that contain no rice. Karyn Seroussi created these when her son became sensitive to rice. If rice is not a problem, use brown rice instead of quinoa. Batter makes good pancakes too.

Ingredients:

1	Banana, mashed
2	Eggs
1/4 Cup	Oil
1/3 Cup	Milk substitute or water
1/2 Cup	Quinoa flour
1/2 Cup	Tapioca starch
1/2 Cup	Potato starch flour
1 tsp.	Xanthan gum
1/3 Cup	Sugar
1/4 tsp.	Salt
2 tsp.	Baking Powder
1/2 tsp.	Cinnamon (optional)
1/4 Cup	Raisins (optional)

Combine dry ingredients and set aside.

Beat together banana, eggs, oil, and milk. Add this mixture to the dry ingredients and combine just until mixed.

Bake at 350 degrees in an oiled muffin tin, for approximately 15 minutes. Use a toothpick to check for doneness.

Maple Rice Bran Muffins

This is another recipe from the U.S. Rice Council. The original recipe calls for chopped apples, but pears can be substituted for those who must avoid apples. The recipe also calls for buttermilk—for a casein-free substitute add 1/2 tsp. of lemon juice to a cup of soy, rice or potato milk For yeast-free diets, alcohol-free maple flavoring could be added to 100% Pure Vegetable Glycerin. Since yeast-free children get so few treats, you might consider baking these muffins in colorful baking papers, and calling them cupcakes!

Ingredients:

1 3/4 Cups	Rice flour
1/4 Cup	Rice bran (can be found in health food stores)
1 TBL.	Baking powder
1/2 tsp.	Xanthan gum
1/2 tsp.	Baking soda
1/4 tsp.	Salt
1 Cup	Milk substitute, with 1/2 tsp. lemon juice added
2	Eggs (or egg substitute or 4 egg whites)
3 TBL.	Vegetable oil
1/3 Cup	Maple syrup
1 Cup	Chopped apples or pears
1 Cup	Raisins
1 tsp.	Cinnamon

Combine dry ingredients in a large mixing bowl.

Whisk together milk, eggs, oil, and maple syrup in a medium bowl. Stir in raisins and fruit.

Make a well in the center of the flour mixture, pour liquid mixture into the well and stir to combine. Spoon batter into lightly greased muffin cups. Use back of wet spoon to smooth tops.

Bake at 425 over for 18-20 minutes. Cool on wire rack. Makes 12 muffins.

Beth's Blueberry Muffins

This is another of Beth Crowell's recipes. It makes a very light muffin which my children like a lot. See variations that follow—all are excellent!

Ingredients:

1 3/4 Cup	Rice flour
1/2 Cup	Sugar
1 1/2 tsp.	Salt
1 3/4 Cup	Water
2	Eggs
1/2 Cup	Oil
2 Cups	Beechnut® Baby Rice Cereal
1 TBL.+2 tsp.	Baking powder
1-2 Cups	Blueberries (fresh or frozen)

Combine four, sugar and salt. Add water, eggs and oil, and mix well.

Stir together rice cereal and baking powder, and add to the above mixture. Mix well and fold in blueberries.

Fill sprayed or papered muffin tins until almost full, and bake at 400 until golden, 20-25 minutes.

Variations:

Use cranberries and orange zest or extract.

Use fresh, sliced strawberries.

Swirl the batter with your favorite jam—heat it first slightly so it will swirl in.

Use your imagination and add whatever you have on hand!

Blueberry Muffins

I love this recipe, which was given to me several years ago. I recently converted it to a muffin my son can eat, and it is almost as good as the original (I cannot tell a lie—the original was even better!) I think you'll like it too, even without real butter, a Granny Smith apple and whole wheat flour. The diced fruit adds moistness and extra flavor.

Ingredients:

1	Egg
1	Egg white
1 Cup	Milk substitute (a rich milk such as soy or potato works best)
1/2 Cup	Vegetable oil
1	Tart pear, peeled and diced
1 Cup	Fresh blueberries
1/2 tsp.	Cinnamon
2 Cups	GF flour
2 tsp.	Xanthan gum
1/3 Cup	Brown sugar, packed
1 TBL.+1 tsp.	Baking powder
1 tsp.	Salt (optional)

Topping:

1/4 Cup	Brown sugar, packed

| 1/4 Cup | Chopped pecans |
| 1/2 tsp. | Cinnamon |

Preheat oven to 350. Grease bottoms only of muffin tins, or use lightly sprayed baking papers.

Beat eggs; stir in milk, oil and fruit. Stir in cinnamon.

In a separate bowl, combine flour, brown sugar (1/3 Cup), xanthan gum and salt. Stir this mixture into the wet mix until moistened (again, a few lumps are OK). Spoon batter into muffin tins, filling about 2/3 full.

Combine topping ingredients in a small bowl, and sprinkle over the tops of muffins.

Bake for about 20 minutes, or until muffins test done. Remove to wire rack at once.

Tropical Muffins

These muffins resulted from combining several recipes in my files. They're delicious for breakfast or as an afternoon snack.

Ingredients:

2 Cups	GF flour
1/3 Cup	Sugar
2 tsp.	Xanthan gum
3 1/2 tsp.	Baking powder
1/2 tsp.	Salt
3/4 cup	Chocolate chips* (I prefer the mini-chips)
3 TBL.	Dry Milk substitute
3/4 cup	Water
1/3 Cup	Vegetable oil

2	Eggs
1/2 Cup	Coconut (unsweetened with no sulfites)
1 1/2 tsp.	Orange oil (available from Williams-Sonoma) or flavoring

*Chopped, dried fruit would be an excellent substitute for chips. Try pineapple or papaya, to maintain the tropical mood.

In a medium sized bowl, combine dry ingredients. Stir in chips or fruit, and coconut.

In a smaller bowl, whisk together the water, oil, egg and orange flavor until light. Add the wet ingredients to the dry and stir together just until moistened and blended together. Don't over beat—a few lumps are OK.

Grease or spray a 12 muffin tin and fill each 2/3 full with batter.

Bake at 400 for about 15 minutes, rotating the tin back to front midway through baking.

Remove when a toothpick inserted in the center comes out clean. Cool on wire racks.

Jam Muffins

Everyone has eaten some version of this very simple muffin. It looks very plain, but bite into it and you are happily surprised by a jam filled center. Fill the muffin cups carefully, or the jam will poke through and spoil the surprise.

Ingredients:

1 Cup	GF flour
3/4 Cup	Jowar flour (or other GF flour)
2 TBL.	Sugar
2 tsp.	Xanthan gum

2 1/2 tsp.	Baking powder
3/4 tsp.	Salt
1	Egg (beaten)
1 Cup	(or more) Milk substitute
1/3 Cup	Oil
4-5 TBL.	Jam or fruit spread

Mix dry ingredients in one bowl, wet ingredients (except for jam) in another.

Combine the two mixtures until just moistened, do not over beat. If the mixture seems too thick, add a little extra milk.

Oil or spray muffin tins, and fill 1/2 full with batter. Add 1 generous teaspoon jam, then cover the jam with a spoonful of batter. Be sure to fill any empty muffin cups with water—I usually get nine muffins from this recipe.

Bake at 400 for 20-25 minutes or until just brown. Makes approximately 10 muffins.

Sweet Potato Rolls

These rolls are similar to biscuits. They make a nice mid-morning snack, or lunch filler. Don't be put off by the sweet potato—even kids who don't like sweet potatoes will enjoy this little bread. They don't rise much, so make the rounds at least 1/2 " thick.

Ingredients:

1 (large)	Sweet potato, peeled and diced
1/4 Cup	Peanut (or other nut) Butter, smooth
1/4 Cup	Pear juice
3 TBL.	Pure maple syrup

3/4 Cup	Brown rice flour
1 1/4 Cups	GF Flour
2 tsp.	Xanthan gum
2 tsp.	Baking powder
1/2 tsp.	Baking soda
1/4 tsp.	Ground cardamom *or*
1 tsp.	Cinnamon

Steam or microwave the potato until tender, but not mushy. Blend until smooth in food processor or blender. Measure the potato—you will need one cup of the puree. Chill it for 10-15 minutes.

Blend (or process) the potato, along with the nut butter, juice and maple syrup, until smooth.

Sift together remaining ingredients, then work into the potato mixture by hand.

Form dough into a ball and roll out on GF flour covered surface. The dough will be smooth, pliable, and easy to roll out. Roll out to 1/2 " thickness and cut out rolls with a biscuit cutter or the rim of a drinking glass.

Bake on oiled or sprayed cookie sheets at 450 for 15 minutes, or until golden.

Mini Sandwich Rolls

These rolls contain no gluten, rice, dairy, egg or yeast. It's a wonder they're so good! If they are made into large rolls, they can be used for hamburger buns. Smaller ones toast nicely for breakfast or lunch. This is another Seroussi recipe.

Ingredients:

| 1/2 Cup | Oil |

1/2 Cup	Milk substitute
1/2 Cup	Quinoa or chickpea flour
1/2 Cup	Tapioca starch
1/2 Cup	Potato Starch
1 TBL.	Sugar
3 tsp.	Ener-g egg replacer (if egg is not a problem, use 1)
2 tsp.	Xanthan gum
2 tsp.	Baking powder

Preheat oven to 400. Beat together oil and milk substitute.

In a separate bowl mix all dry ingredients. Add liquid to dry mixture and combine until just mixed. Don't over beat.

Bake for about 20-25 minutes in an ungreased muffin tin, or spoon onto a cookie sheet. Don't crowd them as they puff up quite a bit. Bake to golden brown. Store well in airtight container, or freeze.

FP Zucchini Bread

You really need a food processor to make this delicious quick bread. If you do not have one, it will take some elbow grease to grate the zucchini, and a strong electric mixer to blend the batter. With a processor, this recipe is very simple, and turns out two moist breads. Like many quick breads, these are really more like cake than bread.

Ingredients:

1 (Large)	Zucchini
4	Eggs
2 Cups	Sugar

1 Cup	Oil (or 1/2 cup prune puree)
1 tsp.	Vanilla
3 Cups	GF Flour
1 TBL.	Xanthan gum
1 TBL.	Cinnamon
1 tsp.	Salt
1 tsp.	Baking soda
1 tsp.	Baking powder
1 Cup	Chopped walnuts (optional)

Shred zucchini in the food processor. Change to the steel blade and add eggs, sugar, zucchini, oil and vanilla. Mix well.

Mix together dry ingredients and add to the processor bowl, process just until mixed.

Pour into two greased 9" x 5" x 3" loaf pans; bake at 375 for one hour or until breads test done.

Coconut Quick Bread

This is delicious when served with Indian food, and can pass for dessert. It's an unusual bread, and one that you should try out on your family. Tip: toasted coconut improves the flavor of many quick breads—be sure to toast extra. Cool completely and then store airtight.

Ingredients:

1 Cup	Grated coconut (no sulfites)
2 Cups	GF flour
2 tsp.	Xanthan gum
3/4 Cup	Sugar

1 TBL.	Baking powder
1 Cup	Soy or other milk substitute
2	Eggs, beaten
1/4 Cup	Oil
1 tsp.	Vanilla

Spread the coconut on a cookie sheet and toast at 350 until lightly browned. Watch carefully, as coconut burns quickly. It should be light brown—stir once. This will take only 3-5 minutes.

Combine the coconut with the dry ingredients and mix well.

In a separate bowl, mix the wet ingredients and add to dry mixture. Blend well and pour into an oiled 9" x 5" x 3" loaf pan. Bake at 350 for 50-60 minutes, until a toothpick inserted comes out clean and the bread is golden brown.

Pearsauce Bread

The recipe was converted from an old-fashioned applesauce bread recipe. Pearsauce is easy to make (see recipe in Chapter 12) or you can use baby food pears; be sure to find a brand that has no fillers or sugar added. For a less sweet bread, adjust the sugar to suit your taste. This is a good after-school snack. My boys like it with their breakfast.

Ingredients:

1 Cup	GF flour blend
1 Cup	Brown rice flour
1/2 tsp.	Baking powder
1/2 tsp.	Baking soda
2 tsp.	Xanthan gum

1 tsp.	Cinnamon
1/2 Cup	CF Margarine
1 1/2 Cup	Sugar
2	Eggs, lightly beaten
1/2 Cup	Applesauce or pearsauce (use a little more if batter seems too stiff)
1/2 Cup	Milk substitute
1/4 tsp.	Lemon juice OR apple cider vinegar
1 tsp.	Vanilla
1/2 Cup	Chopped walnuts and/or raisins (optional)

Stir together dry ingredients and set aside.

In a large bowl, cream margarine and sugar. Add eggs, fruit sauce and lemon juice.

Alternately add the dry ingredients and the milk to the fruit sauce mixture, then stir in vanilla and any optional ingredients.

Bake in an oiled 9" x 5" loaf pan at 375 for 50-60 minutes, until bread tests done with a toothpick.

Sweet Corn Bread

This corn bread is similar to the version served at Boston Market® restaurants. It can be used for Tamale Pie, but more often I use this batter for regular cornbread or for muffins.

Ingredients:

3/4 Cup	Sugar
1/2 Cup	Oil
2	Eggs, lightly beaten

1 1/2	GF flour (choose Hagman mix or soft rice flour)
1 tsp.	Xanthan gum
3 tsp.	Baking powder
1/8 tsp.	Salt
1 1/2 Cups	Yellow corn meal
1 Cup	Milk substitute

Blend together sugar and oil, then mix in eggs.

In a separate bowl, mix dry ingredients well, then blend them into the egg mixture, alternating with milk.

Bake in a greased loaf pan at 400 for 30 minutes, or until bread tests done. For muffins, check after 15 minutes.

Corn Bread II

This version of corn bread is less sweet. If the maple syrup is exchanged for 1/4 to 1/2 cup of 100% Pure Vegetable Glycerin, this can be eaten on a yeast-free diet. Experiment to get the sweetness to your liking. Remember, the glycerin is much sweeter than sugar.

Ingredients:

2 Cups	Yellow or white Cornmeal
2 Cups	GF flour
2 TBL.	Baking powder
2 tsp.	Xanthan gum
1/2 tsp.	Salt
3/4 Cup	Canola or other oil
3/4 Cup	Pure maple syrup

| 2 Cups | Soy or other milk substitute |

Combine dry ingredients in a medium sized bowl.

In a separate bowl combine remaining ingredients. Add to dry mixture and stir well.

Pour into greased 9" x 13" baking pan and bake about 30 minutes at 350. The bread should test done with a toothpick.

Gluten-Free Tortillas

Many wonderful Mexican recipes call for the use of soft, flour tortillas. Most people switch to corn tortillas, if they cannot eat wheat. But Gluten-Free Pantry customer Elaine Smith missed her flour tortillas so much that she developed a recipe for them, using the French Bread/Pizza mix sold by the company. Use these in the Tortilla Casserole recipe in Chapter 7 if you prefer soft, flour-type tortillas to corn, or if corn is not tolerated. This recipe will not work with regular GF flour—the tortillas become very dry and break when you roll them out.

Ingredients:

2 Cups	Gluten-Free Pantry French Bread/Pizza Mix
2 TBL.	Shortening (Elaine uses Crisco, but CF margarine will do)
1 tsp.	Baking powder
1/2 tsp.	Xanthan gum
1/2 Cup	Water, very hot

Combine the first four ingredients and cut shortening into dry ingredients until crumbly (mixture resembles a pie crust).

Add the hot water and mix until a smooth ball is formed. Invert on a lightly (rice) floured work surface, let rest 5 minutes.

Pinch off golf ball-sized pieces of dough and roll them out into circles 6" to 8" in diameter.

— 182 —

Heat an ungreased griddle to high. Place tortillas on griddle and bake just until a bubble appears in the center of the tortilla. Flip over and cook just until done, less than a minute.

These can be frozen and reheated on a hot griddle or fry pan, but they do not reheat well in a microwave. Makes 10-12 tortillas.

Yeast-Free White Bread

Finding a decent bread for sandwiches and toast is hard enough when you can't use gluten, but add the no yeast restriction and you really have problems. This bread mixes up quickly—it's really just a quick bread but resembles regular bread It is certainly better than any yeast-free, gluten-free bread you can buy, and it is very easy to make.

Ingredients:

2 Cups	GF flour
1 TBL.	Xanthan gum
1 TBL.	Baking powder
1 tsp.	Salt
2 tsp.	Egg replacer (optional)
2 TBL.	Vegetable oil
2	Eggs, slightly beaten
1 1/3 Cups	Water
1 TBL.	Honey (Optional, or use other sweetener such as glycerine)

Preheat oven to 350. Spray 8"x 4" loaf pan, and coat with rice flour.

Combine dry ingredients in bowl and mix with electric beater for approximately 30 seconds.

Combine oil, water, eggs and sweetener, and add to dry ingredients with mixer on slow. Mix only until well combined. Pour batter into prepared pan and bake for 55-60 minutes. Test as for cake, with a toothpick. Should be golden on top and test dry in center.

A Few Yeast Bread Recipes...

When baking with yeast, be sure to use brands that are guaranteed gluten-free, such as Red Star or Saf. When a recipe calls for warm water, it should be warm but not hot. Remember, yeast is a living organism; if it isn't warm enough, the yeast will just lie there, but if it is too hot the yeast will die. If you put a (clean) finger into the water, it should feel quite warm that is, it is above your body temperature of 98.6. But if it is too hot to leave your finger in the water comfortably, it is too hot for the yeast. Some bakers combine one-half boiling water with one-half ice water to achieve this temperature.

Almond Flour Bread

This recipe comes from Beth Hillson. You can grind your own almonds very, very fine, or you can order the Almond Flour from her company, The Gluten-Free Pantry. I have trouble getting almonds as powdery as the flour, so I prefer to buy it. This bread is easily adapted for bread machine use.

Ingredients:

1 1/4 Cups+2 TBL.	White rice flour
3/4 Cup	Potato starch
1/2 Cup	Tapioca starch
3 tsp.	Xanthan gum
1 1/4 Cups	Almond flour

1 Cup	Dry Milk substitute (DariFree works well)
1/2 tsp.	Ascorbic acid (dry Vitamin C)
OR	
1 tsp.	Apple cider vinegar
1/3 Cup	Brown sugar
1 1/2 tsp.	Salt
1 3/4 Cups	Warm water
5 TBL.	CF margarine, melted
2	Eggs, lightly beaten
1 TBL.	Yeast

Preheat oven to 350.

In a large bowl, combine dry ingredients with yeast. Add liquids and beat 2-3 minutes on medium speed until mixture is smooth. It will be quite thick.

Scrape into a lightly oiled 9" x 5" loaf pan. Cover with oiled plastic wrap and let rise in a warm place until the dough comes to the top of the pan.

Bake 40-45 minutes and transfer to a wire rack. Cool completely before slicing.

Bread Machine Method

(For a 1 1/2 or 2 lb. capacity machine)

In a large bowl, combine dry ingredients, except yeast. Combine wet ingredients in a separate container. Add dry, liquid and yeast in the order recommended for your bread machine. If you have a programmable machine, set to one knead cycle and one rise cycle. If your machine isn't programmable, choose the Light setting.

Basic Bread Machine Loaf

This is a very good, basic loaf It makes good sandwiches and toast, and has a nice texture. For a treat, add raisins or other dried fruits (when the machine beeps at you), along with spices such as cinnamon, nutmeg or cardamom. For cinnamon raisin bread, use a Tablespoon cinnamon for good flavor and a dark color.

Ingredients:

1 1/2 tsp.	Yeast
1 1/2 Cups	White rice flour (or GF flour mix)
3/4 Cup	Brown rice flour (or Jowar flour)
2 tsp.	Xanthan gum
1 tsp.	Salt
2 TBL.	Sugar
1/3 Cup	Dry milk substitute (DariFree or soy milk powder work well)
2	Eggs (large)
3 TBL.	CF margarine, melted (or vegetable oil)
1 tsp.	Apple cider vinegar
1 Cup	Water, warm

Mix all dry ingredients in a large bowl. Mix in eggs, shortening, vinegar and water. Stir together just to mix, then place in the oiled bread machine pan. Use the Light setting or set programmable machines to one knead and one rise cycle.

Marci's Soft White Bread and Rolls

An enterprising mom of a GF kid devised this recipe. The first time I used it, I formed the dough into rolls. I gasped when they came out of the oven, because they looked exactly like the fancy round rolls served at very good restaurants. Then to my shock (and great disappointment), they began to sink until completely deflated! Other bakers had this experience too, until one experienced baker suggested increasing the oven temperature to 400. This versatile dough can also be used for pizzas, hamburger and hot dog buns, and soft pretzels. NOTE: the bread will work in a bread machine, but has a nicer texture when made in the oven. It looks like a lot of trouble, but if you have a good mixer it can be put together very quickly. You can also make a large batch of dry ingredients (except for yeast) and store in an airtight container. Later, scoop out about five cups of the dry mix and proceed with the recipe. Don't be afraid of the long list of ingredients.

Ingredients:

2 Cups	White rice flour
2 Cups	Tapioca starch
1/4 Cup	Sugar
4 (liberal) tsp.	Xanthan gum
2/3 Cup	Dried DariFree milk substitute
1 1/2 tsp.	Salt
2 tsp.	Sugar
1/2 Cup	Warm water
2 pkg.	Red Star yeast (2 pkg. = 4 tsp.)
4 TBL.	CF margarine or Oil
1 tsp.	White rice vinegar (or apple cider vinegar)
1 1/2 Cups	Water

3   Eggs (or 4 tsp. Egg Replacer mixed with 1/2 Cup water)

Combine the first six ingredients in a large bowl.

Add 2 tsp. sugar to the 1/2 cup warm water, then add yeast. Let stand and 'proof' for 5-10 minutes.

Mix shortening, vinegar, 1 1/2 Cups water, then beat in the eggs.

Add the shortening mixture, then the yeast mixture to the dry ingredients. If necessary, add more water until dough is soft enough to beat.

Beat at high speed for 2-3 minutes, then add a small amount of rice flour until it is firm enough to work with.

NOTE: This dough is extremely soft; if it is too sticky to work with, keep your hands moistened with water or spray them with cooking spray. Keep some tapioca starch nearby for your work surface. Knead by hand for 3-5 minutes. Work in a little more tapioca if necessary.

Heat oven to 400. Grease your baking sheets or pans with cooking spray. You can bake in loaf pans (2) or form the dough as you like—for rolls and buns, use an orange-sized ball of dough.

You can also shape hot dog or hamburger buns or flatten disks for pizza. Mound dough into a larger round for a larger peasant-style loaf, or stretch it out to form an Italian style bread. Place on oiled or sprayed baking sheets, and let rise in a warm spot, covered with sprayed plastic wrap. (Note: if you are in a hurry, this dough can be baked without waiting for it to rise.)

This dough rises fast, so keep a close eye on it! It doubles in size very quickly.

Before baking, make horizontal slits on the tops of your loaves (use a sharp knife, and don't cut deeply into the loaf). Sprinkle some tapioca starch on the top, which looks great and prevents over browning. Alternatively, you can brush on beaten egg yolk thinned with water and sprinkle with sesame or caraway seeds. (Egg replacer and water works too.)

Bake breads for 50-60 minutes. The outside should be golden brown, but be sure the inside is cooked. To test, pick up a bread and tap the bottom. It should sound hollow. If it isn't done, but is already brown, cover the breads with foil and continue baking for a few minutes, testing for doneness every 3-5 minutes.

For pizza shells, bake only about 10 minutes. Cool and freeze. Defrost and top as needed, and bake until toppings are done and the crust is brown. If baking a pizza from fresh (unbaked) dough, brush it with canola oil, add toppings, and bake for 20-25 minutes.

Be sure to use DariFree for this recipe.

GF Pecan Wild Rice Bread

This bread recipe, another from Beth Hillson's files, is similar to the Pecan Rice bread sold at health food stores. As you would expect, it is quite a bit better coming from your oven. If you can't find wild rice flour, you can order it from the Gluten-Free Pantry or other catalogs. For the pecans, you can buy pieces (which are cheaper than whole nuts) and chop fine. I have used pecan meal, ordered from the King Arthur Flour company.

Ingredients:

1 1/3 Cups+1 TBL.	White rice flour
3/4 Cup	Potato starch
1/2 Cup	Cornstarch (use arrowroot if corn isn't tolerated)

1/2 Cup	Dry milk substitute (Ener-g's Nut Quik would be good)
3/4 Cup	Wild rice flour
1/3 Cup	Chopped, toasted pecans (or pecan meal)
1 TBL.	Xanthan gum
1 tsp.	Salt
3 TBL.	Brown sugar, firmly packed
1 tsp.	Cider vinegar or white rice vinegar
1 3/4 Cups	Warm water
4 TBL.	CF margarine, melted
2	Eggs, lightly beaten
1	Egg white, lightly beaten
1 TBL.	Dry yeast

Oven Method

Preheat oven to 375, and lightly oil a 9" x 5" loaf pan.

In a large bowl, combine dry ingredients and yeast. Mix well.

Combine liquids and add to dry ingredients. Beat at medium speed for 3 minutes, using a heavy duty hand held or stand mixer. Dough should be thick and smooth.

Scrape into prepared pan and cover with oiled plastic wrap. Let rise in a warm place until dough reaches the top of the pan. Remove wrap and bake for 40 minutes or until brown and hollow sounding when tapped. Turn onto a wire rack to cool completely before slicing.

Leftover slices may be wrapped and frozen.

Bread Machine Method

Combine dry ingredient except for yeast, and mix well. Combine liquids in a large bowl. Add dry ingredients, liquids and yeast in order suggested by your bread machine instructions. Use white bread and medium crust settings. During the first kneading cycle, open the lid and help mix the dough with a rubber spatula. If dough seems dry or crumbly, add water, 1 Tablespoon at a time until mixture is smooth and moist. Dough should be the consistency of soft clay.

Remove bread promptly after baking cycle ends. If your machine is programmable, use one rise and one knead cycle.

Crispy Walnut Crackers

Beth Hillson shared this recipe too—she developed it after tiring of having to turn down requests for good cracker recipes. The secret to this recipe's success is to roll out the dough as thinly as possible. According to Beth, "It's the difference between a crispy cracker and a jaw breaker."

Ingredients:

4 TBL.	CF margarine
1/2 Cup	Soy or rice milk
2 1/4 tsp.	Dry yeast
3/4 Cup	White rice flour
1/4 Cup	Cornstarch or tapioca starch
1/4 Cup	Potato starch
1 1/2 tsp.	Xanthan gum
1/3 Cup	Walnuts, toasted, finely ground, then measured*
2 tsp.	Olive oil

Kosher salt

Preheat oven to 350.

Melt margarine in a small saucepan and cool slightly. Warm the milk and add the margarine, either on the stovetop or preferably using the microwave. Do not make this mixture HOT.

Stir in yeast and 1 Tablespoon rice flour until dissolved. Let sit until the yeast begins to foam.

Combine remaining rice flour, cornstarch, potato starch, xanthan gum, salt and nuts. Add milk mixture and beat until well blended. Mixture will be crumbly.

Using fingertips, work the dough, adding a teaspoon of warm water at a time (up to 1 1/2 Tablespoons), until dough can be pressed into a ball. Allow dough to rest, covered, in a warm place for 15 minutes.

Spray the back of an 11" x 17" baking sheet with vegetable spray. Set dough on center of sheet and press and roll dough until it reaches the edges of the pan. To prevent stacking, cover dough with oiled plastic wrap and press the roller over the top. Lift the plastic occasionally, to smooth out any winkles in the dough.

Trim edges and cut into squares. Brush with olive oil, prick with a fork, and sprinkle with Kosher salt. Bake for 15 minutes. Turn pan to allow even baking, and bake ten minutes more or until tops are brown. Remove and cool, then store in an airtight container. The crackers keep for five days, and may be frozen.

Makes 24-30 crackers.

* 1/3 cup ground almonds may be substituted.

GF New England Pumpkin Rolls

This recipe was created when celiac Kathy McDermid refused to go through another Thanksgiving without this old family favorite. She spent months working on the recipe, and what follows is the result of that patient process. Kathy can now enjoy New England style pumpkin rolls with the rest of her family, and since she has generously shared her recipe, you can too! They are slightly sweet and very tasty.

Ingredients:

1 1/2 Cups	Rice flour
1/2 Cup	Bean flour
1 Cup	Tapioca Starch flour
1/2 Cup	Brown sugar
1/2 tsp.	Salt
1 tsp.	Ginger
1/4 tsp.	Nutmeg
1/4 tsp.	Cinnamon
1/8 tsp.	Allspice
1/8 tsp.	Cloves
3 tsp.	Xanthan gum
2 TBL.	Egg white powder
2/3 Cup	Dry milk powder
2 tsp.	Unflavored gelatin
2 tsp.	Egg replacer
1/4 Cup	CF margarine, melted
1/2 Cup	Canned pumpkin
1 1/2 Cups	Warm water
2 TBL.	Quick rise yeast
2 TBL.	Sugar
1 tsp.	Apple cider vinegar

Combine the first 15 (dry) ingredients in the mixing bowl of a heavy-duty mixer. Mix on low (the stir setting if your mixer has one) while preparing the rest of the ingredients.

Mix the margarine and pumpkin in a small bowl and set aside.

Mix together the water, yeast and 2 TBL. sugar and let stand until foamy.

Add the yeast mixture, pumpkin mixture and vinegar to the dry ingredients. Continue to beat on low until slightly mixed. Stop mixer and scrape the sides of the bowl, then beat on high for 3-4 minutes. The dough should look like a smooth, thick frosting.

While this is beating, spray 2 muffin tins with a non-stick cooking spray. Divide the dough evenly between the tins, filling each 1/2 full. Smooth out the dough with a spoon that is dipped in water.

Let rise in a warm place (covered with sprayed plastic wrap) until doubled, about 20-30 minutes.

Preheat oven to 350 while dough is rising. Bake for about 10 minutes or until lightly browned.

Remove from pans to cool on a wire rack.

Depending on size you'll get 18 to 24 rolls.

NOTES

Chapter 9
Ethnic and Holiday Foods

GF and CF cooking can be a real trial around the holidays. With a little imagination and a little luck you can probably continue to carry on family food traditions. Since I was raised in a Jewish home, when I think of holiday food I think of special treats served for Rosh Hashanah, Hanukah, Purim and Passover. Many recipes for these holidays are favorites at our house. But I hope you will find some recipes here appropriate for your family too. I am also including some unusual recipes made in other countries. Don't forget that you can modify many of your own family's traditional foods.

I. SAVORY HOLIDAY FARE

Matzo Balls (K'neidlach)

Matzo balls are light airy dumplings made, traditionally, at Passover. They are always served floating in a flavorful chicken soup. Matzo, however, is made from wheat flour. I couldn't bear the thought of a Passover seder with no matzo balls, and was complaining about it to my mother. She remembered that years ago, some women had made their matzo balls from Cream of Wheat® cereal. I had never heard of that before, but tried it, using rice cereal. After a few trials, I determined that the roasted baby rice cereal found at the health food store made the best matzo balls. A tradition was born (or reborn).

Ingredients:

1/2 Cup	Roasted baby rice cereal (be sure there are no fillers added)
Pinch	Salt
1	Egg
1/2 tsp.	Baking powder
1 TBL.	Oil

Mix all ingredients in a bowl, combining well. Cover the bowl with plastic wrap and let rest in the refrigerator for at least 20 minutes. Bring a large pot of water to boil.

With wet or oiled hands, form the mixture in small balls and drop them into the boiling liquid.

Boil, covered, for 30-40 minutes. When done the balls will float to the top of the pot. Remove cooked matzo balls with a slotted spoon. Place one to three matzo balls in each bowl, and ladle in homemade soup.

Matzo balls expand to several times their original size—do not make balls larger than walnuts, or you will have grapefruit sized matzo balls!

Chicken Soup

In addition to being good for cold and flu sufferers, chicken soup is delicious. Served with GF noodles or matzo balls it is a wonderful way to start a holiday meal, or any meal for that matter. I also love chicken soup with cooked kasha (buckwheat groats). The vegetables in the soup add flavor and nutrition, but by the time the flavor has been cooked into the soup, they are quite mushy.

Ingredients:

1	Stewing chicken (use the largest you can fit into your pot)
1	Onion, chopped
1	Clove garlic, minced
2	Large carrots, peeled
1	Parsnip, peeled but left whole
2	Stalks celery, strings removed and chopped
2-3	Sprigs of fresh parsley
	Salt & Pepper
	Water
1 qt.	GF canned chicken broth, optional

Rinse chicken thoroughly then place in pot and cover with water. Add about 2 teaspoons salt and bring to a boil. (Be sure to include the giblets.)

Let the chicken cook for about 20 minutes, skimming the foam off the surface of the water as it collects. When very little foam is collecting on the surface, add the other ingredients to the pot.

Lower the heat and simmer the soup for approximately 2 1/2 hours, checking occasionally to make sure there is enough liquid. If needed, add water or canned chicken broth.

Taste and correct seasonings, then strain the broth carefully and return the clear soup to the pot.

Return some of the cooked chicken to the soup, if desired, and increase the volume by adding more canned broth if necessary. Add some freshly chopped carrot and celery and cook for another 30 minutes, until the vegetables are tender but not mushy.

Refrigerate the soup until the fat congeals on top. Skim fat off with a spoon. Reheat soup before serving. Matzo balls, GF noodles or kasha may be served with the soup, but should be cooked separately. Place these in the bowl, then ladle soup to cover.

Note: When my mother wants an especially wonderful soup, she makes what she calls Double Chicken Soup. For this soup, she makes the chicken soup and strains it carefully. She then uses the broth (instead of water) to cook a second chicken, prepared as above. Soup prepared this way is so rich it is nearly brown, and is particularly flavorful.

Variation: For a child who is extremely reactive to foods and pigments, a white version of the soup can be made by omitting the carrots and parsley and adding 4 stalks of bok choy cabbage (white part only).

Unchicken Soup

For people who can't eat chicken, or who are vegetarians, you can make a version of this soup without the chicken. It is very tasty, and like the soups made with chicken, leftover broth adds flavor and nutrition when cooking rice and other grains.

To make this soup, bring 8 quarts of water to boil in a large pot. Add all the vegetable ingredients listed for chicken soup, but double the quantity of each. Include the parsley and the bok choy (green and white parts).

Cook until the broth has taken on the color and flavor of the ingredients. The vegetables should be very soft.

Strain the broth and return it to the pot. Correct the seasonings, and add a freshly chopped carrot and celery. Cook gently until the carrot and celery pieces are soft, but not mushy.

Remove from heat and stir in 1/4-1/2 teaspoon turmeric, which gives the soup a yellow coloring.

All the soups freeze well.

Sweet Noodle Kugel

This casserole is on the sweet side, but it is always served as a side dish, usually with a meat. It's a nice change from the usual potatoes, noodles or rice dishes.

Ingredients:

1/2 lb.	Cooked GF noodles
3	Eggs
2	Apples, grated (could use pears)
1/2 Cup	Raisins
2/3 Cup	Sugar
1 tsp.	Cinnamon
1/4 Cup	Oil

Grease a 9" x 9" pan. Combine all ingredients in a bowl and mix very well. Pour into prepared pan and smooth with a knife or the back of a spoon.

Bake at 350 45-60 minutes, just until the top is firm and the edges light brown.

VARIATION: Sweet rice Kugel is made by substituting 2-3 Cups cooked rice for the noodles.

Chickpea Snack

This is a tasty and crunchy snack. Since the beans are high in protein, you get a little more than the usual empty calories in savory snacks. For a milder snack, omit the chili and cayenne powders.

Ingredients:

2 TBL.	Sugar
1/2 tsp.	Ground cumin
1/2 tsp.	Chili powder
1/2 tsp.	Paprika
1/4 tsp.	Ground coriander
1/8 tsp.	Cayenne pepper
1/8 tsp.	Salt
2 Cups	Chickpeas, cooked (if using canned, rinse well and drain)
2 tsp.	Vegetable oil

In a large bowl toss together all the ingredients except the oil.

Heat the oil in a heavy 10" skillet for about 1 minute, over moderately high heat. Add the chickpeas and cook, shaking the pan frequently, until dry and crispy. This takes approximately 7 minutes.

Use a slotted spoon to transfer the chickpeas to a paper towel-lined wire rack. Cool completely and store in airtight containers for up to a week.

Falafel

Falafel is sold everywhere in Israel, but especially in the Arab market, where falafel wagons are as common as hot dog vendors in New York. On the streets, falafels are usually stuffed into pita bread, sandwich-style, and covered with enough hot sauce to make you go back and buy that (expensive) imported soda. In Middle Eastern restaurants in this country, they are generally served on a plate, with pita or other flat bread on the side. Add some hummus and/or baba ganoush and you have a wonderful Middle Eastern meal.

Ingredients:

2 Cups	Chickpeas, cooked (drain and rinse well if using canned beans)
1	Onion, chopped
1-2	Cloves of garlic, minced or put through a garlic press
1	Sprig of fresh parsley, minced
1 1/2 tsp.	Coriander
3 tsp.	Cumin
1 tsp.	Cayenne pepper (less for milder falafel)
1 tsp.	Salt
1/2 Cup	Water
1/2 Cup	(approx.) Soy or other heavy GF flour (e.g. brown rice, Jowar, quinoa)
1/2 Cup	Oil (for frying)

Process chickpeas in blender or food processor until smooth, along with 1/2 Cup water. Add the other ingredients (except for oil) and blend well.

Add just enough GF flour to form a dough. With wet hands, form into small balls, the size of a large walnut.

Fry in heated oil, until brown and crispy on all sides. Keep falafel moving in the pot, or they'll stick (they sink at first!). Remove to a paper towel-lined plate and blot excess oil with additional paper towels. Serve with flat bread (e.g. tortillas or Chapatis) and tahini sauce, which has been thinned with lemon juice and hot sauce. Serve immediately if possible.

Baba Ghanoush

Even people who swear they do not like eggplant enjoy this dish. It can be used as a sandwich spread or a dip. It is best scooped up and eaten with a flat bread.

Ingredients:

1	Eggplant, medium sized
2 cloves	Garlic (more if desired)
1/4 Cup	Freshly squeezed lemon juice
1/4 Cup	Tahini (available at most groceries and health food stores)
	Salt & pepper to taste

Preheat oven to 350. Lightly grease the outside of the eggplant, and bake on a sprayed cookie sheet until very tender, around 30 minutes, depending on the size of the eggplant. It is OK if the outside of the eggplant chars a little, but be sure to turn it several times during baking.

When the eggplant has cooled, cut it in half and scoop out the inside. Add the other ingredients to the eggplant, and puree, either in a food processor or blender. I usually put all the ingredients in a bowl and use my Braun Multipractic; this incredibly handy tool is a hand held blender, especially useful when the volume of a dish would require blending in several batches.

Process until quite smooth—you will still see some of the seeds from the eggplant but that is fine. Serve warm or (more commonly) at room temperature.

Hummus

This is the wonderful, high protein partner of baba ghanoush. Serve chilled or at room temperature.

Ingredients:

1 onion	Peeled and minced
2 cloves	Garlic, minced
1 TBL.	Olive oil
1 16oz. can	Chickpeas, drained and well-rinsed
1/2 Cup	Freshly squeezed lemon juice
1/4 Cup	Tahini
1-2	Green olives, large
	Salt, pepper, paprika to taste

Saute the onion and garlic until soft. Remove from heat.

Using a blender or food processor, puree the chickpeas with all other ingredients (except paprika).

Place in a serving bowl, and swirl decoratively with the back of a spoon. Sprinkle with a little paprika. Chill. To be truly authentic, place a little olive oil around the edges of the bowl before serving. Serve chilled or at room temperature.

Indian Flat Breads (Chapatis)

If your family ever eats curries or other Indian foods, this flat bread will complement the meal perfectly. Devised by the mother of an Indian celiac, it is very close to the real thing. Even if your family doesn't like Indian food, the bread makes a nice change of pace, is gluten and yeast-free and is easy to make on top of your stove. You may need to find an Indo-Pak grocery store to get some of these ingredients—such stores contain many unusual products you may want to try, and they nearly always carry Jowar flour. If you can't find cilantro, you might want to grow it in your garden or in a window box. It makes a wonderful addition to Mexican foods, as well as to Indian dishes.

Ingredients:

2 Cups	Rice flour
1/2 Cup	Water, boiling
1 tsp.	Curry leaves, chopped (these are not spicy)
3 TBL.	Chopped, fresh cilantro (many groceries carry this herb)
3 tsp.	Green chilies, minced (canned chilies are very mild)
1/2 Cup	Coarsely powdered roasted peanuts (optional)
1/2 tsp.	Salt
2 TBL.	CF margarine, softened
1-2 TBL.	Ghee (clarified butter, found in Indo-Pak stores) or Oil

Mix flour with boiling water, curry leaves, cilantro, chilies. salt and peanuts (if desired).

Add salt and the softened margarine. Knead into a firm dough.

Divide dough into 8-10 balls and cover them with a damp tea towel or plastic wrap.

Heat a skillet to medium high and sprinkle some rice flour on a clean work surface. Working with one ball at a time, flatten into a thin circle. To be perfectly authentic, use your hands, but if this is hard for you a small rolling pin will do. Keep other dough balls covered while working.

Cook one at a time in a heavy skillet. When one side is dry, flip it over to cook the other side.

When slightly golden drizzle with a few drops of oil or melted ghee (Indian clarified butter, which is generally casein-free). Flip again so that the bottom also gets some fat.

Pathiri

This is another bread served with Indian food, but it is also delicious with any soups, stews or meat. Because Pathiri has a rice base, it is possible to make very authentic breads with only a few modifications.

Ingredients:

1 Cup	Rice flour
1/2 Cup	Water, boiling
1 TBL.	Vegetable oil
1/2 Cup	Coconut milk (canned is fine)

Place the flour in a large bowl and add the boiling water in a steady, slow stream. Stir constantly while adding the water, with a large wooden spoon.

Allow the dough to cool enough to handle comfortably. Then knead the dough on a rice flour covered surface, working in the oil as you knead. The dough is finished when it is very smooth—this takes about 10 minutes of kneading.

Divide dough into 12 pieces, and roll each to form a smooth ball. Grease your hands if the dough is too sticky to work with. Keep dough covered with plastic wrap while you work, rolling each into a 6" round. Dust rounds with rice flour to prevent sticking to each other.

Heat a heavy skillet or griddle over medium heat. Add the rounds, one at a time, and fry on each side until little bubbles or spots begin to form. This takes only 20-30 seconds.

Brush baked Pathiri with coconut milk, fold each in half and keep warm until serving.

Pad Thai

This delicious noodle dish is a staple of Thai restaurants. If your family likes peanut butter, and noodles, you'll probably have a hit on your hands. Although peanuts are traditional, there's no reason another nut and nut butter wouldn't do. If nuts are not tolerated, you could replace the nut butter with tahini.

Ingredients:

1/4 Cup	Peanut butter
3 Cups	Water
7 oz.	Thin rice noodles (also called rice sticks)
2 TBL.	Vegetable oil
1	Clove garlic, minced
1 tsp.	Fresh ginger, minced
2	Scallions, finely chopped
2 Cups	Shredded bok choy or Chinese cabbage
2 tsp.	Wheat-free tamari sauce
1/8 tsp.	Pepper
	Chopped roasted peanuts for garnish (if desired)

Spoon peanut butter into a small dish and set aside.

Bring water to a boil. Add noodles and cook approximately 5 minutes or until the noodles are soft. Use the boiling water, a Tablespoon at a time, to thin the peanut butter until it can be poured. Drain noodles and set aside.

Heat oil in a wok or large skillet over moderate heat. Add garlic, scallions and ginger and stir fry for approximately 2 minutes. Add cabbage or bok choy and stir fry approximately 4 minutes. The vegetables should be tender, but still crispy.

Add the noodles and thinned peanut butter to the wok. Add pepper to taste. Stir fry until heated through and garnish with peanuts if desired. Serve immediately.

Picadillo

I have no idea how authentic this Mexican recipe is. I do know, however, that almost everyone who tries it loves it. I have served it for family dinners and for company; it is always a big hit.

Ingredients:

1 lb.	Ground meat (preferably ground sirloin)
2	Tomatoes, chopped (drained, canned tomatoes can be used)
1	Onion, minced
1/2 tsp.	Cumin
1 tsp.	Sugar
1 tsp.	Salt
2 TBL.	Apple cider vinegar
1/2 tsp.	Ground cloves
1 tsp.	Cinnamon
1	Clove garlic, minced
1/2 Cup	White raisins
1/2 Cup	Slivered almonds
	Pepper (to taste)

Brown meat and drain well. Add chopped onion and continue cooking until the onions are soft.

Add all ingredients except for almonds. Stir well and simmer over low heat for 20-30 minutes. Be careful not to burn it, and if necessary, add a few Tablespoons water.

Spoon into a serving dish and top with almonds. Serve with rice or cornbread.

HINT: Decrease the spices if you want a milder dish.

Corn Fritters

Masarepa is pre-cooked, white cornmeal. Goya brand makes it, so it can often be found at the regular supermarket. It can be used to make these fritters, or for native American corn puddings. If I am serving these for breakfast in place of pancakes, I use white grape juice or pear juice instead of water. I drizzle a little honey on top, and Sam thinks they are great. Use water or a little CF milk to make these as a savory side dish.

Ingredients:

1 Cup	Masarepa
1 1/2 - 2 Cups	Water, CF milk, or juice
2 TBL.	Honey, optional
Oil	For frying

To masarepa, add water orifice and mix until the consistency is that of very thick pancake batter. Fry in very hot oil, until golden brown on both sides.

Empanadas

*Empanadas are made in both Central and South American countries; typically they are filled with meat, but are good with any filling you think your family would enjoy. In her wonderful book, **Still Life With Menu Cookbook** Mollie Katzen suggests* *filling empanadas with bananas and cheese. For a savory filling, add 1 brown onion and ground beef. Process it until almost smooth, then add spices and moisten with a little salsa.*

Ingredients:

2 Cups	GF flour
2 tsp.	Xanthan gum
1 tsp.	Salt
1 Cup (approx.)	Water

Combine flour, xanthan gum and salt in a large bowl, and make a well in the center. Pour in water and stir until well combined. Work with hands if necessary. Knead by hand on a rice floured surface until smooth, about 5 minutes. (Use just enough water to be able to gather dough into a ball. It may take as little as 3/4 cup, or as much as a full cup.)

Divide dough into 8 pieces and knead each into a ball. Flatten the dough balls and roll each to a 5" diameter. Place a Tablespoon filling in the center of each round. Brush the edges of the circle with water, then fold in half, forming a half moon shape. Crimp with fork to seal well.

Repeat for the other 7 empanadas.

Arrange empanadas on a sprayed cookie sheet and brush with melted CF margarine or egg yolk beaten with a Tablespoon water. Bake at 375 for 12-15 minutes. Serve hot.

(If you prefer, fry empanadas, 5 minutes on each side, in margarine.)

Dahl

Dahl is a wonderful side dish very common in Indian cuisine. There are thousands of variations, probably because there are so many types of lentils. Recently, I had the best dahl I have ever tasted at a local Indian restaurant, but I could not get the chef to reveal his secret. I offer a simpler version, which is excellent with any curry or other spicy food.

Ingredients:

8 oz.	Dried red lentils (available at Indo-Pak groceries)
1	Onion (large), chopped
1 tsp.	Ginger
3 Cups	Hot water
1 1/2 TBL.	Ghee, or CF margarine
2	Cloves garlic, minced
1/2 tsp.	Turmeric
	Salt, to taste
1/2 tsp.	Garam masala (a spice mixture found in Indo-Pak groceries)

Wash and pick over lentils, removing any small stones that may have been missed by processing equipment.

Heat fat and fry onion, garlic and ginger. Add turmeric and stir until vegetables are well coated.

Add the lentils and stir well. Fry for approximately 2 minutes.

Add the hot water and bring to a boil. Reduce to a simmer, cover, and cook 15-20 minutes until lentils are soft but not fully cooked. Add salt and garam masala and mix well.

Continue cooking until the dahl has the consistency of porridge. Sprinkle top with extra garam masala and serve.

Variation: Any color lentil will work. White, yellow and red lentils are commonly used; red lentils are often used because they cook so quickly.

Almond Chicken

This recipe isn't authentically Chinese, but it's a nice way to prepare chicken. If your family eats as much chicken as mine does, you will welcome anything a bit different.

Ingredients:

2	Chicken breasts, skinned, boned and sliced thinly*
2 TBL.	Oil
1	Onion, thinly sliced
1 Cup	Celery, chopped
1 Cup	Water chestnuts, drained
5 oz.	Bamboo shoots, drained
2 Cups	GF Chicken broth (check can label or use homemade)
2 TBL.	GF Soy or Tamari Sauce
2 TBL.	Corn starch (or arrowroot starch)
1 tsp.	Sugar (optional)
1/4 Cup	Cold water
1/4 Cup	Almond slivers (toasted)
	Salt

Spread almond slivers on an ungreased cookie sheet, in a single layer. Toast at 300, stirring occasionally, until light brown. Watch the nuts carefully—they can go from brown to black very quickly.

Heat oil in a heavy skillet and saute sliced chicken until it loses its raw appearance, about 2-3 minutes.

Add onion and celery and cook for minutes (covered) before adding water chestnuts, bamboo shoots, chicken broth and GF soy sauce.

In a small bowl, blend sugar, and cornstarch in the cold water. Stir to dissolve the starch. Pour this mixture over the chicken and cook until thick, stirring constantly. Add salt to taste.

Garnish with toasted almonds and serve over rice.

*It is much easier to slice the chicken thinly if the meat is partially frozen.

Sweet and Sour Meatballs

I didn't much like meatballs when I was a child, but when I discovered that they were a favorite for both my boys, I began to cook them. I was very surprised to find that I like them too! This recipe is particularly tasty, and note the grownup variation that follows. For small children, make small meatballs—they will be more readily eaten. These are usually made with ground beef but if you are cutting down on fat use ground turkey.

Ingredients:

2 lb.	Ground beef
1	Onion, chopped very fine
1 TBL.	Garlic, minced
3	Eggs, beaten
1/4 Cup	GF bread crumb mixture* (see recipe in Chapter 7)
1/4 Cup	Water
1 tsp.	Salt
1 Cup	Water
1 32 oz. Can	GF tomato sauce

1 Can	Water
6 oz. Can	Tomato paste plus 1 can of water
1/2 Cup	Brown sugar
4 TBL.	Lemon juice (preferably fresh)
	Salt & pepper to taste

Mix the first seven ingredients and shape into meatballs.

Combine the rest of the ingredients in a large pot and bring to a boil. Lower the heat and drop the meatballs into the sauce. Simmer for approximately 1 hour. Adjust the seasoning to your taste (making it either sweeter or more sour.)

Serve with rice or GF noodles.

*In some parts of Eastern Europe, cooked rice is used as the binder rather than bread crumbs.

Variation:

For the adults at your table, a minor adjustment makes this a more interesting and traditional dish. While the sauce is coming to a boil, bring a second pot of water to a boil. Remove the core of a medium sized head of cabbage. Place the cabbage in the boiling water and cook for about 5 minutes, or until the outer leaves are starting to come away from the head. Remove the cabbage and place it in a colander under cold running water. Work the leaves off carefully. If inner leaves don't come free easily, return the head to the boiling water for a few more minutes.

Place a cabbage leaf on the counter, with the spine of the leaf pointing towards you. Place some of the meatball mixture at the spine, and roll up the leaf to contain the meat. Fold sides of cabbage under the cabbage roll, tucking them under as smoothly as possible (it doesn't have to be perfect!). Carefully place each filled leaf in a Dutch Oven or other wide bottomed pot. Put the smaller, plain (kids) meatballs in too, after the cabbage rolls are all in the pan. Carefully ladle the hot sauce over the meatballs and cabbage rolls. The sauce should cover the meat. Cook at a slow boil for 45 minutes to an hour, depending on the size of the meatballs. (Or, cover and cook at 350 for an hour—be sure the pot is oven proof.)

If there are more leaves than meatballs, toss them into the sauce too. They are very tasty for the cabbage lovers you are serving.

Vegetarian Variation:

The cabbage rolls can be used to make a vegetarian dish too. Instead of a meat filling, fill the cabbage leaves with a mixture of cooked rice and chopped mushrooms, or any vegetable you like, and cook in the sauce for 20 minutes, or until everything has warmed through and taken on the flavor of the sauce.

Potato Pancakes (Latkes)

Often served on Hanukah, potato latkes are good with chicken or meat. Like large Tator Tots®, only better, they are too good to make only once a year. Most grocery stores stock potato pancake mixes in the Kosher section. They are fairly good, but unfortunately nearly all brands add sulfites to the potatoes, so read labels carefully. Since the sulfite is intended to keep the potato white, it's a little silly—latkes are brown when cooked anyway!

Ingredients:

3	Potatoes, peeled
2	Eggs
Pinch	Salt
1/4 Cup	Ground Hol-Grain rice crackers or creamed rice cereal

Oil for frying

Peel and grate potatoes. Squeeze out as much liquid as possible from the potatoes.

Add the eggs, salt and enough of the crumbs so the mixture is stiff enough to form into patties.

Heat oil for a few minutes. Form lathes with wet hands. Fry until golden and crispy on all sides.

Potato Kugel

This is another good side dish. Although it is most often served during Passover, it goes well with any light dinner and is a good way to cook potatoes when you are tired of all the usual sides. Potato Kugel can also be made from latkes mixe, but watch for sulfites.

Ingredients:

6	Medium sized potatoes, peeled
2	Eggs
1/2 Cup	GF flour
1/2 tsp.	Baking powder
1 1/2 tsp.	Salt
1/8 tsp.	Pepper
1	Onion, finely chopped
1/4 Cup	CF margarine

Grate the potatoes and squeeze out as much of the liquid as you can. Add the eggs and mix well.

Sift together the dry ingredients, and add to the potatoes.

Heat margarine in a skillet and saute onion until it is very soft and light brown. Add the onions to the potatoes and stir well.

Pour mixture into a greased, 8" square baking pan. Bake at 350 until the kugel is brown and crispy at the edge, about one hour. Cut kugel into small squares for serving.

Twice-Wild Turkey Stuffing

Most stuffing recipes call for bread, cubed or crumbs. You can certainly use GF bread for this purpose, but there are other ways to stuff a turkey that don't require bread at all. If you prefer, make these stuffings in a casserole rather than inside the bird.

Ingredients:

1/2 Cup	Mixed, dried wild mushrooms
2/3 Cup	Wild rice
2 Cups	Onions, chopped
1 tsp.	CF margarine
1 Cup	Celery, finely chopped
4 TBL.	Salt
1/4 Cup	Cooking sherry
	Generous pinch of: thyme, oregano, marjoram, black pepper

Cover the mushrooms with warm water for at least 30 minutes. Remove from water and squeeze out as much excess liquid as possible. Chop well.

Rinse wild rice in cold water. Bring 3 cups water to a boil, add salt and rice. Return to a boil for 25 minutes, stirring occasionally. Drain well and set aside.

Saute onions and celery in margarine until slightly softened. Remove from heat, add remaining ingredients and mix well. Stuff the bird at once and roast.

Kasha Stuffing

Whenever my birthday falls on a Thursday, it is also Thanksgiving. The first time this happened, I was quite small. Breaking with our usual tradition of Thanksgiving at our house, we instead ate at the home of an aunt and uncle. To this day I remember that the turkey was stuffed with kasha—my all time favorite grain, and that my aunt made a cake for me in the shape of a lamb. I have no idea how my aunt made her stuffing, but this should work if you too love kasha.

Ingredients:

2 Cups	Kasha, whole or coarse grain
2	Eggs, lightly beaten
2 TBL.	Olive oil or CF margarine
4 Cups	GF Chicken or vegetable broth
1/4 Cup	Cooking sherry or another dry wine
1-2	Cloves garlic
2	Onions, chopped
1/4 Cup	Pecans, chopped (optional)
	Giblets

Bring broth to a boil. While broth is heating, stir beaten eggs into the kasha, then cook in a large, deep pan over medium high heat until each grain is separate. Stir carefully to prevent burning and to break apart any clumps of kasha.

Pour boiling broth into the pan, standing back (it will spatter) as you do so. Lower the heat, cover the pan and simmer for approximately 20 minutes or until the broth is absorbed and the kasha is fluffy.

In sauce pan, saute the turkey giblets, onions and garlic until soft. Add to the kasha, then add wine and pecans, if desired.

Mix well, making sure the mixture is well moistened. Stuff the bird with this mixture, taking care to cover the turkey cavity completely with the turkey skin.

The stuffing will dry out if exposed to the oven heat.

II. HOLIDAY SWEETS

Spritz Cookies

My maternal grandmother, Bubby Mary, was a wonderful baker. Much of what I know about baking I learned from her. My mother often dropped me off to spend an afternoon with Bubby, and we always baked something together. She loved to make Spritz cookies, and always used a cookie press to make them look fancy. Without gluten, however, the dough is too soft to put through a cookie press. Instead, I use a pastry bag filled with a large star tip (#6). Pastry bags and tips are sold in stores that carry cake decorating supplies, and in the baking section of most supermarkets. These are perfect for Christmas time, and always find their way into the teachers' baskets I prepare.

Ingredients:

3/4 Cup	Sugar
1 Cup (2 sticks)	CF margarine (room temperature)
1	Egg
1 tsp.	Almond flavoring (I use Frontier® alcohol-free flavorings)
1 tsp.	Vanilla flavoring (Frontier® or use vanilla sugar)
2 Cups	GF flour mix
1/2 Cup	Almond flour (available from the G-F Pantry)
Pinch	Salt (optional)

Using an electric mixer, cream together sugar and margarine until fluffy. Add the egg and flavorings; beat until well blended.

On low speed, gradually add the flours and salt and mix until incorporated.

Place dough in the pastry bag (already fitted with star tip) and fill about halfway. (If you overfill your pastry bag dough will squirt out the top, making a real mess.) Line baking sheets with parchment, and hold pastry bag at a 90 angle from the sheet. Squeeze out desired amount of dough to make a star shape, or lower the angle of the bag slightly and move in a circular direction to make a rosette. Make cookies about 1 3/4" diameter.

For the best shape, hold the tip very close to (but not touching) the sheet. Squeeze firmly until the cookie is the size you want, and then lift the tip straight up to finish.

Decorate the cookies with whatever you want and whatever your family tolerates. You could use glace cherries and other fruits, pearl sugar, sprinkles (use in moderation due to the artificial colors and starches), coconut or even chips. Granulated sugar can be colored with a few drops of concentrated fruit juice (see description in Chapter 8) but this must be done in advance to allow time for drying.

Bake at 375 in the center of the oven for 10-12 minutes. Rotate sheet midway through baking, and if you are using two sheets at once, rotate and exchange top to bottom as well. Cool on racks and store in airtight containers. These freeze well if wrapped tightly.

Gingerbread People

What could be sweeter than little gingerbread folk? I usually make mine in a variety of sizes, and often stick a small cookie hand on the hand of the large Mommy cookie. I even have a tiny boy and girl cutter, these get pressed across the front of the Mommy cookie, and her arms are folded around the baby.

Little girl cookies hold the tiny ones as dolls, and little boy cookies are baked, perched upon the Dad cookies' shoulders. It may be hard to picture, but when decorated with royal icing, they are quite lovely. This recipe comes by way of Karyn Seroussi. I have also used recipes adapted from old favorites.

Ingredients:

2/3 Cup	Brown rice flour
1/3 Cup	Sweet rice flour
1/3 Cup	Tapioca starch
1 TBL.	Cinnamon
1 tsp.	Ginger (use more for a cookie with a real ginger bite)
2 tsp.	Xanthan gum
1 tsp.	Baking soda
1/2 tsp.	Salt
1/4 Cup	Sugar
1/4 Cup	Oil
1/4 Cup	Molasses
2 TBL.	Water

Combine dry ingredients in a large bowl and then add the oil, molasses and water.

Mix well. adding more tapioca starch as needed to make a soft dough that can be kneaded.

Roll out on a tapioca floured board to a thickness of 1/4". Cut out with gingerbread people cutters, dipping cutters into tapioca starch after each use.

Bake in a preheated 350 oven on ungreased cookie sheets for approximately 14 minutes.

Remove from pan while cookies are hot; cool on a wire rack. Cookies will be slightly chewy.

Bubby Mary's Carrot Ring

Bubby often served this carrot ring with dinner, in place of potatoes or another starch. It is almost rich and sweet enough to serve as dessert. My sister and I were crazy about this dish, and Bubby often made it just for us. The GF version isn't quite as good as the carrot rings I remember from childhood, but it is very tasty and sure to be liked by all.

Ingredients:

1/2 Cup	Light brown sugar, packed
1 Cup	CF margarine
2 Cups	Grated carrots
1	Egg, beaten with 1 TBL. water
1 1/2 Cups	GF flour (or 1 cup GF flour and 1/2 Cup brown rice or jowar)
2 tsp.	Xanthan gum
1/2 tsp.	Baking soda
1/2 tsp.	Salt
1/2 tsp.	Baking powder
1/2 tsp.	Nutmeg
1/2 tsp.	Cinnamon

Cream sugar and margarine, add carrots and when well mixed, beat in egg.

Sift together dry ingredients and add to creamed mixture.

Place in a ring mold, cover, and refrigerate for at least 2 hours.

Bake at 350 about 35 minutes or until golden brown.

Mandel Bread

My mother and her mother always made these twice-baked cookies for Hanukah. Their recipe adapted very easily to gluten-free flour, so they are again a Hanukah staple for us.

Ingredients

6	Eggs
1/2 cup	Oil
1 Cup	Sugar
1 tsp.	Baking powder
3 Cups	GF flour
1 tsp.	Salt
1 tsp.	Vanilla
	Cinnamon and sugar

Beat eggs, oil and sugar. Add baking powder, flour, salt and vanilla (it will be a stiff batter).

Shape into 2-3 thin loaves and place on a greased cookie sheet.

Bake 30 minutes at 375 (until light brown).

Slice on the diagonal while still warm. Lay slices on cut side, sprinkle with cinnamon and sugar mixture. Toast in a 300 degree oven until crispy and brown, about 45 minutes.

For fancier cookies, divide the dough into four pieces. The resulting cookies will be much smaller and will look nicer.

Hamentashen

This is a treat served for the Jewish holiday of Purim. They have become very popular however, are often available year-round in bakeries and stores on the east coast. The cookies are very soft (unless you over-bake) and they freeze well. If made small, they look nice enough for a fancy cool tray. One of the traditional fillings is made with poppy seed, which I avoid when baking for children. (See recipe for Sesame Fingers in Chapter 10 for a discussion of poppy seeds.)

Ingredients

4	Eggs
1 Cup	Vegetable oil
1/4 tsp.	Salt
4 1/2 Cups	GF flour
1 tsp.	Vanilla
1 1/2 Cups	Sugar
2 tsp.	Xanthan Gum
4 tsp.	Baking powder

Suggested fillings:

Cherry, apricot or other pie type fillings or fruit jam. Most stores carry various brands. Check ingredients carefully, since many of these fillings contain starch. Most use tapioca, which is fine, but make sure the label states the source of the starch.

Cream sugar and oil, then add eggs and blend well. Stir in vanilla.

Mix together dry ingredients and add to wet. Roll out on GF floured surface. Cut into 2 1/2" circles.

Add 1 teaspoon filling and moisten edges of dough with water. Bring together sides of circle to form a triangle, with the filling peeking through the middle. Pinch edges of dough to hold shape.

Bake on a lightly greased sheet at 350 for 10-15 minutes.

Honey Cake

It is traditional to eat foods sweetened with honey for the Jewish New Year (Rosh Hashanah) so we may have a sweet new year. Honey cake is very common at this time of year, and lends itself to GF flours very well.

Ingredients:

3	Eggs
1 Cup	Sugar
1 Cup	Honey
1/2 Cup	Oil
1 Cup	Apricot preserves
2 tsp.	Baking soda
3/4 Cup	Black coffee, cooled
1	Apple, grated (may be replaced with pear)
1	Juice and Grated rind of one orange
3 Cups	GF flour
3 tsp.	Xanthan gum
1 tsp.	Salt
1 tsp.	Cinnamon
1 tsp.	Allspice
1 tsp.	Nutmeg
1 tsp.	Ginger
2 Cups	Walnuts, chopped (optional)
1/2 Cup	Raisins (optional)

Beat sugar and honey on medium speed. Add eggs, one at a time, then add preserves, oil and spices. Dissolve the baking soda in coffee and add to mixture. Mix in the nuts, salt, flour, xanthan gum, juice and apple.

Line the bottom of two 9" x 5" loaf pans with foil or parchment, then grease and flour. Pour batter into the pans and bake at 350 for 20 minutes. Reduce the heat to 325 and bake for an additional 40 minutes. Cool cakes on wire racks, then loosen with a knife and turn out onto serving plate. The extra cake freezes well.

Pesach Banana Cake

Because flour is forbidden on Passover (Pesach), this is a good time of year to look for recipes and ingredients. Many grocery stores carry lots of foods available only for Passover, which are acceptable for the GF/CF diet. If you find something your family enjoys, stock up. Passover is a spring holiday, so check your calendar and watch for these special foods. This cake tastes very light. For a more festive cake, serve with a little warmed chocolate syrup drizzled on top (see recipe in Chapter 12).

Ingredients:

7	Eggs, separated
1 Cup	Sugar
1/4 tsp.	Salt
1 Cup	Mashed bananas (or banana baby food)
3/4 Cup	Potato starch

Preheat oven to 350 degrees.

Beat eggs whites untill stiff, set aside.

In an electric mixer, beat egg yolks well. Add the sugar and salt slowly, beating until the mixture becomes thick and lemony. Add bananas and potato starch while beating and combine well. Mix in a few spoonfuls of beaten egg whites to lighten mixture (by hand).

Add remaining egg whites and fold in gently, losing as little air as possible.

Bake in an ungreased, 10" tube pan for 45 minutes. Invert and let cool completely. (Parchment circles, precut to fit tube pans, are available at good kitchen supply stores. These are very helpful for any kind of sponge cake, which must be baked in an ungreased pan.)

TIP: If you are using a stand mixer, there is no need to clean the beaters or bowl after you have beaten the egg whites. Simply do the whites first and transfer them to another bowl until needed.

Chapter 10
Cookies

June Cleaver may not have been your mom, but no doubt cookies and milk were a common after school snack. Although we all eat too much sugar, most parents would hesitate banning cookies completely from their children's diet. Children on special diets can enjoy these treats too. If you are careful with ingredients, most of your favorite recipes can be adapted. In fact, cookie recipes are more forgiving than bread, cake or muffin recipes, so it is hard to go wrong.

For children with special needs, small bites of cookie are often used as primary reinforcers during discrete trial sessions. In fact, cookies are reinforcing for everyone, the ultimate comfort food, especially when eaten warm from the oven. While good GF cookies can be purchased, at over $3.00 a dozen, store bought cookies become an expensive treat. And of course, they just aren't the some as homemade. I always make sure my son's school has a bag of GF cookies or cupcakes in the freezer, for those unexpected occasions when other children are having regular treats. Most schools won't mind tucking a package like that into a corner of their freezer.

This chapter contains some of my son's favorite cookie recipes. You will note that some recipes call for the use of parchment paper. This paper can be found in most groceries, and in any store that sells cake decorating supplies. It saves a lot of grief when you remove cookies from the pan, and will greatly lessen clean-up time. I often lay out cookie sheet sized pieces of parchment, fill them all with cookie dough, and then slide them on to the sheets for baking. When a batch comes out of the oven, I slide the sheet right on to the cooling rack, and slide on a new sheet of dough for immediate baking.

A word about servings. Most cookbooks tell you how many cookies the recipe will make. I have not included the number of cookies to expect from a given recipe because, no matter how many I expect to get, I never do! It depends entirely on how large you make cookies. I prefer them big so I routinely get a dozen fewer than the recipe number. If you like small cookies, you will get more. In general, a recipe that calls for two cups of flour will yield about two dozen big cookies, three dozen small cookies. If a recipe calls for three or more cups of flour—add another dozen cookies. For bars, you determine how big to cut a brownie or pumpkin square—it's your decision.

You may want to reread the sections on flours and baking techniques in Chapter 5. I recommend you experiment with flours, and with nuts, dried fruits, chips and other add-ins. Use what your family likes. Be creative and experiment. Baking cookies is also a wonderful way to spend time with your child. Even the most destractible child will get interested in this kind of activity—and many a speech or math lesson has been taught while mixing, stirring, measuring and pouring. Little fingers can be taught to crack eggs and little hands are good at stirring. So pull up a stool, tie on the aprons, let the flour fly and make cookies!

NOTE: GF Flour refers to the Hagman blend of rice flour, potato starch and tapioca starch.

Amaretti

Wrap these cookies in 7"squares of tissue paper for a festive look at holidays or parties. Tissue paper now comes in a wide variety of colors and patterns, and seasonal themes are available around the holidays. Kids love unwrapping them to see what's inside!

Ingredients:

1	Egg white
1 tsp.	Almond extract
1 2/3 Cups	Blanched almonds, ground fine*
1 1/2 Cups granulated)	Confectioner's sugar (will NOT work with

Lightly beat egg white and almond extract. Combine almonds and sugar and then mix in wet ingredients to form a paste. Shape mixture into small balls and bake on parchment lined sheets for 15 minutes at 350. Sprinkle with powdered sugar when cookies are baked. Cool on sheets.

*You can use almond flour, available at the Gluten-Free Pantry (see Appendix I) instead of ground almonds.

Chocolate Biscotti

I found some delicious GF chocolate biscotti at the health food store, but they were very expensive. I wanted to duplicate the cookie, so I modified my mother's mandel bread cookies (recipe in Chapter 9) and came up with this delicious facsimile. They're a little more trouble than most, since they are twice-baked, but they are very good and are pretty enough to serve to company. They also make great dunkers whether coffee or milk is the beverage of choice.

Ingredients:

6	Eggs, extra large
1 1/4 Cups	Oil
1 1/2 Cups	Sugar
1/2 tsp.	Salt
2 tsp.	Vanilla
5 Cups	GF flour
1 Cup	Cocoa
6 tsp.	Xanthan gum
2 tsp.	Baking powder
1/2 tsp.	Baking soda
1 Cup	Chopped nuts (optional)

Cream together eggs, oil, sugar, salt, vanilla. In another bowl, sift together dry ingredients and then add to the creamed mixture. Stir in nuts, if desired and tolerated. Chill dough, about an hour.

Divide dough into six portions. Form each into a tube-shaped roll, about 1 1/2" in diameter. Place rolls on greased baking sheet. Bake at 350 degrees for 20-25 minutes.

While still warm, cut the rolls into 1/2" slices (cut slightly on a diagonal for the prettiest cookies). Lay the slices on a flat side, sprinkle with sugar, and toast in a 275 oven for 25 minutes. Turn each slice, sprinkle again and toast for an additional 25 minutes.

The Best GF Chocolate Chip Cookies

I love the chocolate cookie mix sold by The Gluten-Free Pantry. I did not want to depend on having a mix on hand, and of course it is always cheaper to do it yourself. I tinkered around with their basic ingredients and came up with this recipe. They are really wonderful, and while they're not exactly the same as the gluten filled cookie, I have never had any cookie eater complain or even inquire. If tolerated, you can add a cup of chopped nuts. To make chocolate-chocolate chip cookies, replace 1/4 cup of rice flour with 1/2 cup of unsweetened cocoa. These make very soft cookies.

Ingredients:

1 1/2 Cups	White Rice Flour
1 tsp.	Baking soda
1/4 Cup	Potato Starch
1/2 Cup	Sweet Rice Flour
2 tsp.	Xanthan Gum
1/2 tsp.	Baking powder
1 tsp.	Salt
1/2 Cup	Sugar
1/2 Cup	Brown Sugar
1 Cup	CF margarine
2	Eggs
1 tsp.	Vanilla
12 oz.	CF chocolate chips
1 Cup	Walnuts, chopped (optional)

Combine first seven (dry) ingredients in a small bowl. Set aside.

Cream sugars and shortening until well blended. Beat in eggs, one at a time. Add vanilla.

Gradually add flour mixture and mix well. Stir in chips, nuts if desired.

Drop by rounded teaspoons on an ungreased baking sheet. Bake 10-12 minutes in a 375 oven.

Cool on a wire rack. Can also be made into pan cookies by placing in an 8" square pan and baking for 20 minutes or until a toothpick tests dry.

Cut Out Sugar Cookies I

These can be formed with cookie cutters for holidays or other festive occasions. They can be glazed with a mixture of powdered sugar and a few teaspoons milk substitute or fruit juice, to glazing consistency.

Ingredients:

2 1/2 Cups	GF Flour mix
2 tsp.	Xanthan Gum
1 Cup	Sugar
1 Cup	CF Margarine, softened
1	Egg
1 tsp.	GF Baking Powder
2 tsp.	Fruit juice (preferably pear)
1 TBL.	Vanilla

Combine all ingredients and beat until well mixed. Wrap in plastic wrap or seal in a plastic bag and chill until firm. Roll out the dough, half at a time, on a rice floured surface. Cut out with cookie cutters of your choice and place 1" apart on an ungreased sheet. Bake 6-10 minutes at 425 until slightly brown around the edges.

Cut Out Sugar Cookie II

Beth Hillison, the genius behind The Gluten-Free Pantry in Glastonbury, Connecticut contributed this recipe. It is wonderful, as are her many baking mixes! Add cinnamon, nutmeg and ginger for wonderful gingerbread cookies. The cookie dough flour mixture used in this recipe works very well for nearly all cookies. Mix up a big canister and keep it on hand if you are an avid cookie baker (or you are the parent of avid cookie eaters)! Great for Christmas cookies or for a "decorate your own cookie" party.

Ingredients:

1 Cup	CF Margarine
2/3 Cup	Sugar
1	Egg
1 tsp.	Vanilla
2 1/2 Cups	GF cookie flour (recipe follows)
1/2 tsp.	Xanthan Gum
1/2 tsp.	Salt

Cream margarine with sugar until light and fluffy. Add egg and vanilla and beat. In a separate bowl, measure out the gluten-free flour mixture, the xanthan gum and salt. With a fork, combine dry ingredients until well mixed. Add to creamed mixture and beat for one minute.

Chill dough for 2-3 hours or overnight.

Preheat oven to 350, and dust a smooth surface with 1-2 Tablespoons rice flour or cornstarch.

Roll out dough to 1/8" thickness. You can also roll out half the dough at a time between two sheets of plastic wrap or wax paper. Cut out shapes with cookie cutters. Transfer cookies to lightly greased cookie sheets with a spatula. Bake 8 minutes. Cool and frost if desired.

GF COOKIE FLOUR:

1 Cup	Rice flour
3/4 Cup	Sweet rice flour
1/4 Cup	Cornstarch (use arrowroot if corn is not tolerated)
1/2 Cup	Potato starch

FROSTING:

Beat together 2 TBL CF margarine, softened and 1 tsp. vanilla Add 2 Cups powdered sugar and beat.

Add 1 TBL. milk substitute

Keep alternating remaining sugar and milk until consistency is thick and smooth and doesn't drip off the knife. Add more sugar (to 3 cups) and milk (to 3 TBL.) as necessary for proper texture.

Chocolate Krinkles

Just about every cookie cookbook around has a variation on this cookie. It's called everything from Chocolate Crackles to mini-brownies. They do indeed taste like little brownies— chewy and delicious! This is not a spur of the moment recipe though, for it requires a lengthy refrigeration of the dough prior to forming and baking.

Ingredients:

1/2 Stick	CF margarine
3 Squares	Unsweetened chocolate, melted
1 1/2 Cups	Sugar
2	Eggs

1 tsp.	Vanilla
1 1/2 Cups	GF flour mix
1 tsp.	Xanthan Gum
1 1/2 tsp.	Baking Powder
1/4 tsp.	Salt (optional)
	Confectioner's sugar

Cream the margarine until light, then add the sugar and melted chocolate. Mix well. Add the eggs and vanilla. Stir together the dry ingredients and add to the margarine mixture. Mix well, cover and refrigerate for three hours.

Shape dough into balls about 1" in diameter. Roll balls in the powdered sugar and place on greased cookie sheets, leaving 2" between balls. Bake for 10 minutes at 350. Cool on sheet for 5 minutes and then move to wire rack. Be sure to roll in powdered sugar before baking—as cookies spread the sugar forms the crinkled appearance.

Easiest Macaroons

With only three ingredients, what could be simpler? Take care not to burn these, and parchment paper is a must—otherwise they will stick! Mini chocolate chips are a delicious addition to these cookies.

Ingredients:

1 3/4 Cups	Unsweetened coconut, shredded
1/2 Cup	Sugar
1 (or 2)	Egg White(s)

Mix coconut and sugar and add an egg white. Start with one egg white and if it's dry add a second. Batter should be sticky but not runny. Drop by rounded Tablespoons on to a parchment lined cookie sheet. Bake at 350 until light brown, approximately 12 minutes.

Mac Macaroons

Another simple macaroon recipe, this one uses no coconut. Macadamia nuts are well tolerated by most people. They are expensive, but make wonderful additions to baked goods. Watch for sales, or buy them in bulk at health or gourmet shops.

Ingredients:

1 1/2 Cups	Macadamia nuts, ground
1 Cup	Sugar
2	Egg whites
	Salt
	Confectioner's sugar

The nuts should be ground as fine as possible, without turning to a paste. Add some of the sugar to the nuts, and grind in a food processor or blender.

Combine the nuts, remaining sugar, salt and mix well. Add the egg whites and mix into a paste.

Shape the cookies into balls or use a pastry bag (without a tip) to form rosettes. Place on parchment covered baking sheet.

Bake one sheet at a time, in the center of a 325 oven for 18-20 minutes. They should look brown, but should still be chewy. Don't over-bake or you'll burn the bottoms.

Sprinkle with powdered sugar just before serving.

Gingersnaps

This cookie is fragrant and delicious. We like them soft, but if you want some real snap bake them for a little longer. If colors don't cause problems for your child, they can be sprinkled with colored sugar for holidays, or you can color sugar yourself by adding a few drops of natural color (see Chapter 11). White crystal or pearl sugar also add a festive quality.

Ingredients:

3/4 Cup	Shortening (white vegetable shortening is preferable for this cookie)
1 Cup	Sugar
1	Egg
1/4 Cup	Molasses
1 tsp.	Cinnamon
2 Cups	GF flour mix
1 tsp.	Xanthan Gum
1/2 tsp.	Salt
1 tsp.	Ginger (can use more)
1/2 tsp.	Baking soda
	Granulated sugar

Cream shortening and sugar, then add the egg and molasses. Sift and combine dry ingredients and add to creamed mixture. Roll into walnut sized balls, then dredge in granulated sugar. Bake at 350 for 12-15 minutes. Bake 10-12 minutes for soft, chewy cookies, longer for crispy snaps.

Cookies will spread so be sure to space them 2" apart.

Fudgiest Brownies

Every brownie lover falls into one of two camps: those who think that fudgey brownies are best, and those who like cagey brownies. This recipe fills the bill for the first group. They are incredibly fudgey. Serve in very small squares—they are very, very rich.

Ingredients:

2/3 Cup	Sugar
1/3 Cup	CF margarine
2 TBL.	Water
12 oz.	CF chocolate chips (or chopped semi-sweet chocolate)
2	Eggs
1 tsp.	Vanilla
3/4 CUP	GF flour mix
1/4 tsp.	Baking soda
1 tsp.	Xanthan Gum

Combine sugar, margarine and water in a small saucepan and bring just to a boil. Remove from heat and add the chips. Stir until chocolate is melted. Beat in eggs, one at a time. Add vanilla.

Combine remaining ingredients and add to the chocolate mixture. Pour into a greased 9" square pan and bake at 325 for 30-35 minutes. Do not over-bake.

Ronnie's Brownies

My friend Barbara Crooker pointed out that this recipe, originally devised by a college friend of hers, defies my brownie categorization. In Barbara's words, "These brownies are neither cakey nor fudgey, but in between, with that crackly surface that only really great brownies have." If your child cannot eat soy, this is the recipe to choose. I have yet to find a chocolate chip that does not contain dairy or soy lecithin or both. German Sweet Chocolate contains only chocolate, cocoa butter and sugar. I have found that these brownies improve with age—they are much better the second and third day (if they last that long).

Ingredients:

2/3 Cup	CF Margarine
1 Bar	German Sweet Chocolate
2	Eggs
1 Cup	Sugar
1 Cup	Hagman's GF Flour mix
1/2 tsp.	Baking powder
1 tsp.	Xanthan gum
1/4 tsp.	Salt
1 tsp.	Vanilla
1 Cup	Chopped nuts (optional)

Melt margarine and chocolate in microwave or in top of double boiler. Put eggs and sugar in a large bowl, mix, and add the melted chocolate mix. Stir flour, baking powder, salt and xanthan gum together in a small bowl, then add to chocolate mix. Add vanilla and nuts.

Pour into a greased (or sprayed) 8" square pan. Bake for 40 minutes at 325.

Sesame Fingers

Several years ago I created this recipe, using wheat flour and poppy seeds. I was trying to duplicate biscuit that I'd eaten at an expensive gourmet coffee shop. For this version, I use GF flours and changed the seed to sesame. Poppy seed pods contain a naturally occurring latex, and contamination can occur during the harvest. This latex contains morphine-related compounds. I don't know if they could have an actual opioid effect on a child, but it can cause a false positive in a urine drug screening. It seems better to be safe, and the cookies taste very good when made with sesame seeds.

Ingredients:

1/2 Cup	CF Margarine
1/4 Cup	Sugar
1/4 Cup	Brown Sugar, packed
2	Eggs
1 tsp.	Vanilla
2 Cups	GF Flour mix
2 tsp.	Baking powder
1/4 tsp.	Salt (optional)
1/2 Cup	Sesame or poppy seeds
2 tsp.	Xanthan gum
	Additional sesame seeds, for coating Milk substitute

Cream margarine and sugars.

Add eggs and vanilla and blend well. Stir together the dry ingredients and add them to the creamed, mixing well. Then mix in seeds. Roll small pieces of dough into 2" ovals (or fingers), approximately 3/4" thick. Dip in milk substitute and then roll in additional sesame seeds. Place on lightly greased baking sheets.

Bake 15 minutes at 350 or until golden.

Jamie's Awesome Cookies

This recipe lends itself to many variations. Experiment with fruits, spices and nuts. It was created by an Internet friend, Karyn Soroussi, whose extremely food-sensitive child has inspired her to devise many new recipes.

Ingredients:

1	Egg
1/4 Cup	Canola oil
4 oz.	Jar baby fruit (banana or pear)
1 tsp.	Vanilla
1 Cup	Instant brown rice baby cereal
1/4 Cup	Quinoa flour, or chickpea flour
1/4 Cup	Brown sugar
1 tsp.	Baking powder
1 tsp.	Xanthan Gum
1/2 tsp.	Salt (optional)
3/4 tsp.	Cinnamon
1/2 Cup	Golden raisins

Mix egg, oil, fruit and vanilla. In another bowl combine the rest of the ingredients except the raisins. Add dry to wet, then stir in raisins. Drop by teaspoons on to a greased baking sheet.

Bake 10-12 minutes at 350 degrees.

Pumpkin Bars

My friend, Harriet Barnett sent me this recipe. It's very moist but not too sweet, so it makes a good breakfast cake for those who hate to eat breakfast. You can also bake this in a smaller, deeper pan (9"X 13") but you will need to increase baking time slightly.

Ingredients

4	Eggs
1 1/2 Cups	Sugar
1 1/2 Cups	Vegetable oil
1/2 Cup	Applesauce or Baby Pears
16 oz.	Canned pumpkin or squash
1 Cup	Rice flour
1 tsp.	Salt
1 tsp.	Baking powder
1 1/2 tsp.	Cinnamon
1 1/2 tsp.	Nutmeg
1 tsp.	Xanthan gum
3/4 Cup	Chopped nuts (optional)
3/4 Cup	Golden raisins

Beat eggs, sugar, oil, fruits and pumpkin till fluffy. Add the dry ingredients. Mix well and spread batter in a 15" x 10" x 1" jelly roll pan. Bake at 350 for 25-30 minutes.

Meringues

These are lovely cookies—crispy and light as air. You can also stick two together with melted chocolate or thinned jam, for lovely GF petits fours. But be warned—make them on a rainy or humid day and they will degenerate to a sticky, gooey mess. Store in a tight container and do NOT refrigerate or freeze. This recipe also forms the basis of one recipe included in Chapter 11.

Ingredients:

1 Cup	Egg whites (see note)
Pinch	Salt
1/8 tsp.	Cream of Tartar
2 Cups	Sugar

Whip the egg whites and salt in a large (grease-free!) bowl until foamy, then add the Cream of Tartar. Beat until peaks just begin to form. Add sugar gradually and beat until stiff peaks form.

(For chocolate meringues, beat 1/4 cup of unsweetened cocoa into egg whites.)

Use a pastry bag and a Number 4 star tip to pipe the meringues onto a parchment covered sheet.

Pipe in a variety of shapes, if desired, or just in circles. Bake at 250 for 45 minutes or until slightly crisp on the outside. Leave in oven with the door closed several hours or overnight to dry completely.

NOTE: Powdered egg whites are available in most stores, and since you don't need the yolks this is a good way to go. Just follow the directions on the can for reconstituting 1 cup of egg white. If you use real eggs, be sure they are fresh. It will take 6-8 eggs to equal 1 cup of white.

Rice Puffies

I adapted this simple recipe long ago, from one I found on a cereal box. They're not as sweet as my other cookies, but have a satisfying bite. This cookie makes a good addition to a lunch box.

Ingredients

1 Cup	GF flour
2/3 Cup	Sugar
1 tsp.	Xanthan Gum
1 1/2 tsp.	Egg
1/2 Cup	Baking soda
1 tsp.	CF margarine
1 1/2 tsp.	Vanilla
3 Cups	Puffed rice cereal
1/2 Cup	Chocolate chips (optional)

Sift together dry ingredients. Cream butter, sugar and vanilla until light and fluffy, then beat in the egg. Stir in dry ingredients, then cereal and chips. Bake at 350 for 12 minutes or until light brown.

Nut Butter Chippers

Many people are allergic to peanuts. If your child cannot tolerate these legumes try substituting almond, cashew or pistachio butter. All are available at health food stores. If NO nuts are tolerated, try using tahini—a thick, nutty paste made from sesame seeds. You may also try some of the mock peanut butters available through mail order (see Appendix I).

Ingredients:

1/2 Cup	CF margarine
3/4 Cup	Nut Butter
1/2 Cup	Brown sugar, packed

1/2 Cup	Sugar
2	Eggs
1 1/2 Cups	GF Flour Mix
1 tsp.	Baking soda
1/2 tsp.	Baking powder
9 oz.	CF chocolate chips (optional)
1 tsp.	Xanthan gum

Cream margarine with nut butter until soft, then beat in the sugars and eggs. Beat until light; if the mixture seems too heavy add 1-2 Tablespoons water or juice.

Add the dry ingredients and mix well, then stir in chips. Drop dough by rounded teaspoons on to a greased or parchment lined cookie sheet. Flatten slightly with a (wet) fork, making the traditional criss-cross pattern If desired. Bake 12-15 minutes at 350. The center will still be slightly soft.

Keep on sheets for 2 minutes, then move to wire racks.

Aztec Crisps

Aztec Cereal® is available at many health food stores, and is made from the grain amaranth. Some celiac groups suggest avoiding amaranth, but it is not closely related to wheat or other gluten grains, and it has never caused a reactionary my very intolerant son. If peanut butter is not tolerated, try using a different nut butter or tahini.

Ingredients:

1/2 Cup	Sugar
1/4 Cup	Brown sugar (packed)
1/2 Cup	Peanut Butter

1/2 Cup	CF Margarine*
1	Egg (or egg substitute)
1/2 tsp.	Baking powder
1/2 tsp.	Baking soda
4 Cups	Aztec Cereal
6 oz.	GF/CF chocolate chips

Mix first seven ingredients, blending well. Stir in cereal and chips. Shape into balls, and bake, 2" apart on an ungreased cookie sheet. Bake until golden at 325, 10-12 minutes.

I recently made these cookies but forgot to add the margarine. They were delicious!

Spiced Pear Cookies

This was originally made with wheat flour, butter and applesauce. This adaptation is very good. Pearsauce is easy to make (see recipe Chapter 11) and less bland than baby food pears, but either produce a good cookie. If you buy baby fruit, be sure to buy a brand that contains no added sugar, or starches.

Ingredients

1/2 Cup	CF margarine
1/2 Cup	Brown sugar
1/2 Cup	Sugar
1/2 Cup	Pear sauce (or baby pears)
2 Cups	GF flour mix
2 tsp.	Xanthan Gum
1 tsp.	Baking soda
1/2 tsp.	Cinnamon

1/4 tsp.	Ground cloves
1	Egg
1 1/2 tsp.	Salt (optional)
1/2 tsp.	Nutmeg
1 Cup	Golden raisins

Cream margarine and sugars. Add egg and blend well. Add pearsauce to the mixture and blend.

Stir together dry ingredients and add raisins. Add to creamed mixture and blend well.

Drop by teaspoons onto greased sheets and bake 10 minutes at 375. Let cool on baking sheets for 2 minutes, then move to wire racks.

Sugar Sandies

This recipe was adapted from one my mother gave me. When made with wheat flour, they are crispy and light, with a smooth texture. The GF version has a wonderful sandy texture, which was preferred by many tasters who have eaten both versions. If tolerated, you can use a few colored sprinkles for special occasions. These cookies are fragile and won't travel well. Freeze any crumbs or broken cookies, as they can be used in pie crusts and dessert fillings.

Ingredients
1 Cup	CF margarine
2 Cups	Sugar
2	Eggs
1 Cup	Vegetable oil
1/4 tsp.	Salt (optional)

1 tsp.	Vanilla
5 Cups	GF flour
1 TBL.	Xanthan Gum
2 tsp.	Baking soda
2 tsp.	Cream of tartar

Cream margarine and sugar, then add eggs, oil, salt and vanilla. Add the dry ingredients and mix well. Roll dough into small balls and place on ungreased sheet. Flatten with the bottom of a drinking glass that has been dipped in sugar. Bake at 350 for 10-12 minutes.

Optional Icing:

1 Cup Confectioner's sugar, mixed with 2 teaspoons milk substitute and 2 teaspoons corn syrup.

Sweet Pizza

This is a lot of fun at a party or other festive gathering. Strawberry or raspberry jam makes a good 'marinara' for this pizza, however apricot is especially tasty.

Ingredients:

1 Recipe	Cut out Sugar Cookies I or II
1/4 Cup	Jam or fruit butter
1/3 Cup	CF chips
1/3 Cup	Unsweetened coconut (No sulfites)
1 TBL.	Chopped nuts
1 Cup	Dried fruit (e.g. apricots)

Spread the cookie dough onto an ungreased pizza pan (10-12") and press to form a crust. Bake at 300 for 25 minutes.

Spread with jam while still hot and return to oven for 5 minutes. Sprinkle with chips, coconut, dried fruit, and nuts and then cool. Slice into wedges to serve.

Cherry Almond "Mookies"

Beth Hillson of the Gluten-Free Pantry assures me that this cookie brings out the kid in everyone! Tart dried cherries can be found in many health food and gourmet stores. If you own a hydrator, they are easy to dry along with other fruit and vegetables. This saves a lot of money! Be sure to use tart (pie) cherries rather than Bing (or other sweep cherries. The most delicious ones can be ordered from American Spoon Food (see Appendix I.) I have also used Craisins®, sweetened dried cranberries packaged by Ocean Spray, and they were very good. Recently, I made this recipe for a cookie table at a PTA function at my son's school. My husband overheard one parent telling another to "be sure to taste THOSE." So much for needing wheat flour and real butter!

Ingredients:

1 Cup	White rice flour
3/4 Cup	Tapioca Starch
1/4 Cup	Cornstarch, or Potato Starch or Arrowroot Powder
1 tsp.	Xanthan Gum
1/2 tsp.	Salt
1/2 tsp.	Baking soda
1/2 Cup	Applesauce, Prune puree or Pearsauce
4 oz.	Almond paste or Marzipan
2	Eggs (or 4 egg whites), lightly beaten
1/2 Cup	Sugar

1/2 Cup	Brown Sugar, packed
1/2 Cup (1 stick)	CF Margarine at room temperature
3/4 Cup	Dried tart cherries, coarsely chopped
1/2 Cup	Shredded coconut (sulfite-free)

Preheat the oven to 375. Combine the first six ingredients and set aside.

Cream the fruit sauce with the almond paste. Add the eggs.

In a separate bowl beat the butter with the sugars until light and fluffy. Add to the fruit mixture and beat to combine. Fold in the dry mixture and readjust until moistened. Fold in cherries and coconut.

Line baking sheets with parchment paper or aluminum foil. Scoop out dough in heaping teaspoons and set 1" apart on sprayed cookie sheet. Bake 8 minutes or until just lightly browned on the edges. Let cookies cool briefly on pans and then transfer to a wire rack. Cool completely.

Toffee Squares

This is an old recipe that many people have in their files (in one version or another). This one comes by way of Barbara Crooker, who got it from her mother and mother-in-law.

Ingredients:

1/2 lb. (2 sticks)	Unsalted, CF Margarine, softened
1 Cup	Light brown sugar
1 tsp.	Vanilla
1	Egg yolk
2 Cups	GF Flour
8 oz.	Dark chocolate

| 1/2 Cup | Pecans or walnuts |

Cream the margarine with the brown sugar, vanilla and egg yolk. Add the flour and blend.

Spread in a greased jelly roll pan, 12" x 18" and bake at 350 for 20 minutes.

Remove from oven and place chocolate bar on top. After chocolate has melted (from the heat of the crust), spread it with a knife and sprinkle with nuts. Press nuts into the chocolate with the back of a large spoon. Cool and cut into small pieces.

Crispie Treats

These marshmallow treats are everybody's favorite. Be sure to read the ingredients on the crisped rice cereal box carefully; most contain barley malt. Only buy those brands that include no malt at all. Make sure the marshmallows specify corn or tapioca starch rather than modified food starch. If corn is not tolerated, use the recipe in Chapter 12 to make your own marshmallow creme.

Ingredients:

5 Cups	Crisped rice cereal
2 oz.	CF Margarine
1 bag	Marshmallows (or one recipe of homemade marshmallow creme)

In a heavy saucepan melt margarine and marshmallows. Stir well to prevent burning. When the consistency is very loose, stir in the cereal and mix well and quickly.

Press the mixture into a greased 9" x 13" pan. If necessary, spray your hands or the back of a spoon and press to even thickness. Allow to cool and harden completely, then cut into squares with a sharp knife.

Crunchy Crisps

This is a delicious cookie, with lots of crunch. Most groceries and health food stores carry quinoa flakes. They are packaged by the same company that makes the grain itself so if you can find quinoa you will be able to find the flakes. Rice flakes (available from Kinnikinick Foods—see Appendix I) may be substituted.

Ingredients:

1/2 Cup	CF Margarine (use coconut butter if you prefer)
1/4 Cup	Sugar
1/2 Cup	Brown sugar
1	Egg
1/2 tsp.	Vanilla
1 Cup	GF flour
2 tsp.	Xanthan gum
1/2 tsp.	Baking soda
1/2 tsp.	Baking powder
1/4 tsp.	Salt
1 Cup	Quinoa flakes
1 Cup	GF rice crisped cereal (be sure there is no malt!)
1/2 Cup	Coconut (no sulfites)

Cream the margarine and sugars, then beat in egg and vanilla.

Mix together the dry ingredients and add them to the creamed mixture. Drop by teaspoons onto greased or parchment lined cookie sheets. Bake at 350 for 10 to 12 minutes, or until lightly browned. Cool on sheet for one minute, then remove to wire rack.

Chapter 11
Desserts

When I want to make a cake or pie for a guest, I always try to make it something that we can all eat. I look for recipes that use no flour (or very little) or for something that is easily adapted. Because it isn't always possible, I keep some GF cupcakes in the freezer. Usually though, given a little warning, I can come up with something that everyone can enjoy.

Most of these recipes call for eggs—reread the section on replacing eggs in Chapter 5, and then you may need to experiment. While few recipes in this chapter can be used on a yeast-free diet, some may be converted by using 100% Pure Vegetable Glycerin, or powdered stevia.

In general, however, desserts are desserts, and usually require some sugar. But take heart—unlike the GF diet, most times yeast-free is not a lifelong regimen.

Remember: When I specify GF Flour that means the Hagman blend. You may experiment with other flours and blends, of course, adding more or less liquid as needed.

"Farfel Cake"

This is not a cake, nor does it contain farfel (matzo crumbs). It is a recipe given to me years ago by a grad school friend, Michele Blum. I am often asked for this recipe—and it is so easy I'm almost embarrassed to share it! This pat-in crust can be used for any fruit pie. Hint: be sure to use a large enough pan (9"-10") so your crust will be thin.

Ingredients:

1/2 Cup	CF Margarine (a stick)
1/2 Cup	Sugar
1 TBL.	Vegetable oil
2	Eggs
2 tsp.	Vanilla
2 Cups	GF flour
2 tsp.	Xanthan gum
2 tsp.	Baking powder

Cream margarine, sugar and oil. Add the other ingredients and mix well. Divide the dough (it will be soft) in half. Wrap one half in plastic and place in refrigerator until firm. Pat the other half into the bottom and sides of a 10" pie or quiche pan. Fill with a jar of good quality jam or with a favorite fruit pie or tart filling.

Grate the second half of the dough on top of the filling, forming a streusel topping and bake for 1 hour at 350 or until golden brown.

Variation: For a simple, mock linzer torte, exchange one 1/4 Cup of the flour for 1/4 Cup almond or pecan meal, and use raspberry jam to fill. You will get raves, I promise.

Chocolate Cake

This is a lovely, moist cake that will do very nicely as a birthday cake for anyone in the family. I tinkered with an old recipe from my files and came up with this on the first try. Buy mayonnaise from the health food store—there are many brands available made from various oils (such as canola); some use no eggs, and many contain no additives. You should be able to find one that is suitable for your family. This recipe also makes terrific cupcakes.

Ingredients:

2 Cups	GF Flour
2/3 Cup	Unsweetened Cocoa
2 tsp.	Xanthan Gum
1 tsp.	Baking soda
1/2 tsp.	Baking powder
3	Eggs
1 2/3 Cups	Sugar
1 tsp.	Vanilla
1 Cup	Mayonnaise
1 1/3 Cups	Water

Combine flour, cocoa, xanthan gum, baking powder and baking soda in a medium sized bowl.

With an electric mixer, beat eggs, sugar and vanilla until smooth. Beat at high speed until light (approximately 3 minutes). Reduce speed to low and beat in mayonnaise. Alternately beat in flour mixture and water.

Grease and flour two 8" or 9" round pans for layer cake, or a 9" x 13" sheet cake pan.

Bake at 350 for 25-30 minutes until a cake tester comes out clean. Cupcakes take 15-20 minutes. Cool in pans for 10 minutes, then transfer to wire racks. Frost and fill, if desired, when completely cool. For an unfrosted cake, place confectioner's sugar in a sieve; sprinkle on cooled cake (it is best to use a 9" x 13" pan if you don't plan to frost).

Chocolate Frosting

Beat together until smooth:

1/2 Cup	CF magazine, softened
1 Cup	Confectioner's sugar
2/3 Cup	Unsweetened Cocoa
2 TBL.	Milk substitute (use more or less to achieve spreading consistency)

Chocolate Torte

The easiest way to bake without gluten is to find recipes that don't call for any in the first place. Each year, Barbara Crooker makes this for her son David's birthday. Barbara always lets a little casein slip through for this cake, because it is so wonderful when made with real butter. If your child can't tolerate any casein (many cannot) use CF margarine. Without flour, this cake requires eggs—don't attempt this one with egg substitute.

Ingredients:

8 oz.	Semisweet or Bittersweet chocolate (dairy free)
3 oz.	Butter or CF margarine
1 1/4 Cups	Sugar
5	Eggs (large)
1 pint	Raspberries or strawberries (if berries are not in season, use canned (drained) mandarin oranges)
1 TBL.	Sugar

Grease a 9" round pan, line with waxed paper or a parchment circle; grease the paper too. If using a springform pan (with removable bottom) fit a double thickness of aluminum foil around the outside of the pan to prevent leaking.

Melt the chocolate in a double boiler (chocolate can be melted in a microwave, but it burns quickly and must be stirred often). When chocolate is almost completely melted, add the butter and stir until both are melted and evenly blended. Set aside to cool this mixture slightly, and bring water to boil in a large pot or kettle.

Add sugar to the chocolate mixture. In a separate bowl beat eggs until foamy, and then beat eggs into the chocolate. Be sure the chocolate is no longer hot, or you run the risk of cooking your eggs. Beat just until the mixture is completely blended.

Pour cake batter into your prepared pan. Place the boiling water in a pan large enough to hold your cake pan, and put the cake pan inside this water bath.

Bake cake at 350 for 90 minutes. Remove the cake pan from the water bath and cool for one hour on a wire rack or to room temperature. Refrigerate cake for at least two hours once cooled.

Loosen the sides of the cake with a wet knife and invert the cake onto a plate or wire rack and (if made in a springform pan, remove sides of pan, and once inverted, remove pan bottom and paper). Invert once more, this time directly onto your serving plate.

Decorate with one-half pint of the berries. You may want to sieve some powdered sugar on first, and then place berries along border or in whatever pattern desired.

Optional: puree remaining 1/2 pint of berries with 1 TBL. sugar to make a fruit sauce. Either pass the sauce separately, or place a large dollop of sauce on each plate and put the cake on top.

Serve small slices this is a very rich dessert!

Pineapple Velvet Cake

An Internet friend, Lynne Davis, created this recipe. Pineapple juice is tolerated by most people, and adds a lovely flavor without being overpowering. People who don't know the name of this cake rarely guess that pineapple juice is an ingredient. This is my standard birthday cake and cupcake recipe. Lynne uses a simple pineapple glaze, which is delicious. For birthdays I use either a CF butter cream frosting or a fluffy boiled icing; both can be piped into decorative borders, stars or words. By placing little toys or ornaments on the cake it is festive and fits with the party theme. Recipes for both icing options follow. This terrific cake is so versatile—be sure to read all the notes that follow.

Ingredients:

2 1/2 Cups	GF flour mix
1 tsp.	Baking soda
2 tsp.	Xanthan gum
3 tsp.	Baking powder
1/2 tsp.	Salt
4 tsp.	Eggs
1 Cup	Canola (or other vegetable) oil
1 2/3 Cups	Sugar
2 tsp.	Fresh lemon juice
1 Cup	Unsweetened pineapple juice

Combine the first five ingredients and set aside.

With an electric mixer, blend eggs, oil, sugar and lemon juice. Beat well so oil is completely emulsified, and the mixture is light and lemony looking.

Turn beater to low, and add flour mixture and pineapple juice, alternating.

Pour batter into greased and floured tins (a 9" x 13" pan, two 9" round cake pans, or cupcake tins). Bake at 350 for 25-30 minutes for cakes, 15-20 minutes for cupcakes.

Lynne's Easy Pineapple Glaze

| 3 TBL. | Pineapple juice |
| 1 1/2 Cups | Confectioner's sugar |

Heat juice in saucepan or microwave until very hot. Whisk in powdered sugar until it is a smooth, thick, runny liquid. Place cooled cake on wire rack, set on a large sheet of aluminum foil. Pour glaze over the top of the cake, starting at the middle. Use a frosting knife to guide the glaze to the edges of the cake if necessary; cover sides quickly (while glaze is still hot and runny) if desired. You can also just let the glaze drip attractively down the sides without trying to cover the sides.

NOTE: As stated above, this is a very versatile recipe. It has a lovely texture, and can be modified for nearly any flavor you want. Simply replace the juice in the recipe with another flavor juice, or with liquid milk substitute (to start with a more neutral base). For example, to make a maple cake you might replace some of the sugar with pure, granulated maple sugar (available at gourmet shops and through mail order). Then use natural maple flavoring in place of the vanilla, and flavor the frosting to suit the cake you have made.

Fluffy White Frosting

1 1/2 Cups	Sugar
1/3 Cup	Water
2	Egg whites (I prefer to use dehydrated whites to eliminate any concern over salmonella, and because it is less wasteful.)
1/4 tsp.	Cream of tartar
Pinch	Salt
1 tsp.	Vanilla (or other flavoring)

Boil water in the bottom of a double boiler (or a large, heat-proof bowl which fits over a saucepan). While water is heating, combine the sugar, water, salt, egg whites and cream of tartar in the top of the double boiler (or large bowl). Beat with electric mixer on low for 30 seconds to combine.

Set pan or bowl over the boiling water (be sure that the bottom does not touch the boiling water). Beat on high speed, for 7 minutes. The volume will have greatly increased. Remove from heat, add vanilla and beat for 2 more minutes until firm and glossy. Frost and/or till completely cooled cake. Over time, frosting gets harder on the outside. It tastes somewhat like marshmallow cream and is still delicious.

Using Natural Colorings

White frosting is shiny and pretty, but sometimes children would really like some COLOR on their cake. This is still possible, even if you are avoiding all artificial colors and preservatives.

The icing can be colored with a small amount of cherry or raspberry juice for pink icing. The tiniest bit of beet juice, not enough to impart a flavor, will make an intense reddish pink.

Blueberry juice makes a light blue to purple icing.

Regular juices made for drinking contain far too much water to be used for this purpose.

You need something really bright and intense; I suggest buying bags of frozen (unsweetened) fruits. Because there are so many uses for these fruits (e.g. adding to pancakes, muffins etc.) it isn't wasteful.

Place the frozen fruit in a colander, suspended over a glass bowl or pie pan. As the fruit thaws you will collect approximately 1 to 3 oz. of deeply colored juice. Since it takes so little juice to use as a coloring, the extra can be stored in small glass jars and frozen for later use. For beets, use a fork to prick a few holes in the vegetable. Cook for just a few minutes so they are a bit soft (the microwave works well) and when cool enough to handle, squeeze them over a glass bowl. (Wear plastic gloves or your hands will also be pink!) Only a tiny amount is needed, so it won't impart a beet flavoring to the icing. Use your imagination and experiment with other naturally occurring colors. (Look for art books which use natural pigments—some are not appropriate for conscription, but many are.)

Leftover Frosting:

If you have any leftover frosting, do not throw it away! Heat your oven to 250 and line baking sheets with parchment paper. Use a pastry tube and a large star tip to pipe the extra frosting onto the paper. Bake until dry and just starting to color (don't let them brown). This usually takes about 30 minutes. Turn off oven and leave the cookies inside for several hours, to dry completely. Voila! Delicious crunchy meringue cookies.

Buttercream Frosting

"OK, OK enough already." I hear you say! Not quite. Here is another frosting to use on either the Pineapple Velvet Cake or the Chocolate Cake. This is the easiest of all frostings to

decorate with, and has enough structure to pipe into roses or other decorative items. This frosting will stay soft, and is very versatile. You can use maple, lemon or any other flavoring that suits both your mood and the cake.

Ingredients:

1/2 Cup	CF margarine
1/2 Cup	Solid white vegetable shortening*
1 Lb.	Confectioner's sugar (grind your own if corn isn't tolerated)
1 tsp.	Vanilla
2 TBL.	Milk substitute
2-3 TBL.	Corn syrup (if tolerated)

In a mixer, combine margarine, shortening and vanilla plus any other flavoring used. Beat until very smooth. Add the sugar, one cup at a time, and beat until mixed. Cover the mixer with a towel while adding the sugar—the powder will fly and make a big mess.

Beat for several minutes after all sugar has been added. Beat in milk and add corn syrup to reach spreading consistency. If corn syrup isn't tolerated, use extra milk.

*If white shortening isn't tolerated, use all margarine. The resulting frosting will be softer and harder to pipe, but it will taste fine. If there is not suitable margarine you can substitute coconut butter (see Appendix I for source).

Any extra frosting may be frozen for later use.

Remember Twinkies®?

You can make your own version of these (beloved by all children) Hostess® treats. To make a GF version of the old standby, bake the Pineapple Velvet Cake in a sheet (jellyroll) pan. When it is completely cool, cut the cake into (Twinkie®-sized) rectangular pieces. Make a slit on the side of each piece with a sharp knife, and fill with Fluffy White Frosting. Alteratively, start at a short end of a Twinkie® and make a hole through its middle with a straw then use a pastry bag and tip to fill.

For an easier, albeit less authentic looking treat, just make cupcakes and use a pastry bag to fill.

Remember, each one has a fairly small amount of the sweet stuff inside, so don't go overboard with filling. For Hostess® Devil's Food Cupcakes, fill chocolate cupcakes instead. Be sure to save a little frosting so you can pipe that famous squiggle on top!

Black Magic Cake

This recipe has something of a history. Mrs. Martha Dunn shared it with the readers of a Celiac news group on the Internet. She got the recipe from her sister, Karen Gorney of Grangeville, Idaho, who got it from her husband's great, great grandmother! The cake has a very smooth texture and if unfrosted can be eaten with the fingers. It has the added benefit of being very easy to put together—definitely a good cake for novice bakers. I predicted this cake would be too sweet and was prepared to cut the sugar; to my surprise it was just right. To bakers everywhere, Mrs. Dunn offers this sage advice: "Don't let the kids dance in the kitchen while you're baking!"

Ingredients:

1 3/4 Cups	White rice flour
3/4 Cup	Unsweetened cocoa
2 Cups	Sugar

2 tsp.	Baking soda
1 tsp.	Baking powder
1/2 Cup	Oil
1 tsp.	Salt
1 1/2 tsp.	Xanthan gum
1 Cup	Black coffee (brewed and cooled-may be decaffeinated)
2	Eggs
1 tsp.	Vanilla
1 Cup	Milk substitute, soured with
1 tsp.	Lemon juice or vinegar

Combine dry ingredients in one bowl and wet ingredients in another bowl.

Combine wet with dry and beat until blended, then pour batter into greased pan(s). Use either a 9" x 13" sheet, or two 9" round cake pans.

Bake at 350 for 35-40 minutes or until a toothpick inserted in the center comes back clean.

This cake would make a very good birthday cake, baked in rounds and frosted with one of the previous recipes. Without frosting, it is an excellent snack cake—with a light sprinkling of powdered sugar you will have a lovely, light cake or a great after school treat.

Apple Cake

When I first moved to New York in 1977, many stores and bakeries carried "Jewish Apple Cake." Although well versed in Jewish baking, I had never heard of such a thing. I still have no clue what makes this kind of cake Jewish. Origins notwithstanding, these cakes are moist and delicious, and are great for those slow starters who won't eat a real breakfast. You can, as always, substitute pears.

Ingredients:

2 Cups	GF flour
1 tsp.	Baking powder
1 1/2 Cups	Sugar
2 tsp.	Xanthan gum
2 tsp.	Cinnamon
1 tsp.	Salt
1/2 Cup	Oil
3	Eggs, lightly beaten
1/2 tsp.	Baking powder
3/4 Cup	Brewed, cold coffee (decaffeinated is fine)
1 1/2 tsp.	Vanilla
2 1/2 Cups	Apples or pears, peeled and sliced
1 Cup	Chopped nuts (Optional)

Dissolve baking soda in the coffee.

Mix dry ingredients in a large mixing bowl; stir in wet ingredients and blend. Add fruit and nuts.

Pour into a greased 9" tube pan. Bake at 350 for 50-60 minutes or until it tests done.

Cool cake for 10 minutes, then invert pan over plate (it may not drop immediately, and if it is stubborn, run a knife gently around the sides of the pan).

Sprinkle with powdered sugar and serve warm or room temperature.

Fruit Cobbler

My sister gave me this recipe years ago and I found it works just as well with the GF flour mixture. To my knowledge, this is the only thing (other than cranberries on Thanksgiving) she cooks. She is lucky that her husband likes to cook and is very good at it. This dessert is perfect for fruit just starting to darken, but too good to throw away. If possible serve it warm from the oven.

Ingredients:

5 Cups	Fruit (berries, sliced pears or apples, plums, peaches etc.)
1/2 Cup	Sugar (use less if the fruit is really sweet and ripe)
2 TBL.	GF flour
1 TBL.	Lemon juice
1 tsp.	Vanilla
1/2 tsp.	Cinnamon

Topping:

1	Egg
1/2 Cup	GF flour
1/2 Cup	Sugar
2 TBL.	CF margarine, melted
1/2 tsp.	Baking powder

Mix fruit with sugar, GF flour, lemon juice, vanilla and cinnamon. Toss until fruit is evenly coated. Place mixture in a 2 Qt. casserole or baking dish. Dot with margarine, if desired.

Mix topping ingredients and spoon onto fruit, covering as much of the fruit mixture as possible (it doesn't have to be perfectly covered).

Place a sheet of aluminum foil on the bottom of your oven—this is very messy! Bake at 375 until topping is golden, approximately 45-50 minutes.

This is delicious on its own, but absolutely wonderful if served warm with ice cream (or sorbet).

If you like a topping with a crumbly texture, add 1/4-1/2 Cup of ground pecans or almonds.

During winter, use apple or pears together with fresh or frozen cranberries. Add a few golden raisins and you have a wonderful dessert.

Rice Pudding

When I was young, my mother always made a baked pudding with leftover rice. I think she was the only one who really liked it, but then she always poured lots of heavy cream over hers! I have always preferred diner-style rice pudding, and my children love it too. It can be made with any kind of raw rice, but brown rice will take longer to cook.

Ingredients:

1/2 Cup	Rice (raw)
2 Cups	Milk substitute (have more ready—it is often needed)
Dash	Salt
2	Eggs
1/2 Cup	Sugar (less if you plan to add raisins or other dried fruit)
1 tsp.	Vanilla
1/2 - 1 Cup	Raisins or other dried fruit (unsulfited)

Bring the milk, rice and salt to a boil in a heavy saucepan.

Cover and simmer over very low heat for at least 20 minutes. Watch this carefully, and stir very often to prevent scorching. Add more milk as necessary to thin and prevent burning.

Beat together the eggs, sugar and vanilla until thick.

Add the egg mixture to the rice and return to the heat; cook 2-3 minutes more, stirring constantly. Remove from heat and add cinnamon and raisins if desired.

Serve warm or cold.

Simplest Pudding

If your children tolerate soy, this is an easy and painless way to get some extra protein into their diet. I saw a mix in the grocery store, which contained little other than cocoa, xanthan gum and sugar. The package directions said to blend with a block of Tofu. I didn't buy the mix, which appeared to be GF but was quite expensive. I went home and tried it, even though I felt fairly certain my children would give it the "thumbs down." Well, surprise! They loved it. Stronger flavors such as chocolate are easier to get by a suspicious child than a milder fruit flavor.

Ingredients:

1 10 oz pkg.	Firm silken tofu (light tofu is fine)
1/4 Cup	Cocoa
3/4 cup	Sugar
1 tsp.	Vanilla
1 tsp.	Xanthan gum

Drain and crumble the tofu, then use a blender or food processor to make a smooth, puree texture. Add cocoa, sugar, xanthan gum and vanilla to the tofu and mix until it is uniformly brown. Spoon into serving dishes and chill.

Pudding Variations:

Chocolate Pie

Double the recipe and spoon it into a baked pie crust. It could also be spooned into a pre-baked meringue or rice crust (see recipes below).

Fruit Pudding

Instead of melted chocolate, you can blend in fresh fruit and a GF flavoring that goes well with the fruit. Bananas are very good, and so are rasberries and peaches.

Pudding Pops

Most groceries carry plastic ice pop molds. To make pudding pops, thin the pudding mixture with some rice or soy milk. Pour into ice pop molds and freeze. These are a real treat for most children.

Pavlovas

*This recipe always reminds me of the Floating Island dessert Katharine Hepburn served to Spencer Tracy in one of my favorite old movies, **Desk Set**. In fact, it is probably very similar, but I prefer the lovely Russian name. The dessert is simply a thin pudding, with little meringue cookies floating in it.*

Ingredients:

2 Dozen (or more)	Meringue cookies (see recipe in Chapter 10), very small
1 Recipe	Lemon pudding (see recipe in Chapter 12)
1/3 Cup	Fresh lemon juice*

| 1 pint | Fresh berries (raspberry, blueberry or strawberry) |

Prepare vanilla pudding from mix as directed in Chapter 12, omitting the vanilla. When pudding is well chilled, thin it with fresh lemon juice, a little at a time, until the consistency of thin custard.

At serving time, spoon 2-3 Tablespoons custard on to each dessert plate, and float 4-6 tiny meringues on top. Garnish with fresh berries.

*If you prefer a vanilla custard, use vanilla flavoring instead of lemon, and thin the custard with milk substitute.

Bolo De Coco

Many nationalities have much more rice in their diets than Americans typically do. These cultures are great sources of recipes without wheat or other gluten grains. This particular recipe comes from Sri Lanka, and required little modification since rice flour is a common ingredient in Sri Lankan cuisine. It is quite different, and very good. If nuts are not tolerated, omit them. It would be a good dessert after any Asian meal.

Ingredients:

3 Cups	Dried, unsulfited coconut
3 Cups	Water
4	Eggs, separated
1/4 tsp.	Cream of tartar
2 Cups	Sugar
2 Cups	Rice flour
1 Cup	GF flour
2 tsp.	Xanthan gum

2 tsp.	Baking powder
1/2 tsp.	Ground cardamom
1/4 tsp.	Cinnamon
1 TBL.	Water*
4 oz.	Raw cashews or blanched almonds, finely chopped

Line a 10" square pan (or two loaf pans) with parchment paper. Spray paper lightly.

Combine water and coconut in blender or food processor. Blend until coconut is finely ground, about 2 minutes. If you have a small blender or food processor, you may have to do this in two batches.

Combine egg yolks, 1 Tablespoon coconut mixture and sugar in a large bowl. Beat until the mixture is well blended. Add the rest of the coconut mixture and beat again until well blended.

Combine the dry ingredients and stir them into the wet mixture, along with the nuts.

Beat the egg whites in a clean bowl until foamy. Add cream of tartar, and continue beating.

Add 1/4 Cup sugar gradually, and beat until stiff peaks form.

Fold the egg whites into the coconut mixture, taking care not to deflate the whites too much.

Pour batter into pan(s) and bake 1 1/4 to 1 1/2 hours until it tests done with a toothpick. Place pan on a wire rack and cool completely before serving.

*In Sri Lanka, rose water would be used instead of plain water. You can use it if you like, but most Americans find rose water flavoring too reminiscent of soap.

Making GF Pies

Neither of my kids care much about pie, but many adults prefer a good pie to cake or cookies.

The problem is, making good GF pie crust is a real challenge. Pie crust just seems to cry for gluten, and it's quite difficult to make a really good one without it. (Recently, The Gluten-Free Pantry and Miss Robens have added pie crust mixes to their mail order offerings.) Sometimes, it's better to use something unusual for a crust (such as rice or meringue) or sticking with a graham cracker or cookie crust. Some pies (e.g. pumpkin) can be baked without any crust at all, by pouring the filling into ramekins and baking without benefit of any flour.

The secret of making a good pie crust was explained to me long ago by Lynn Kutner, a baking instructor at the New York Restaurant School. According to Kutner, there are five essential elements involved in making a light and flaky pie crust. First, fat must be cut into the flour in such a way that it remains distinct and separate from the flour—that is, fats should not be creamed or melted into the dough. To achieve this, you must cut the fat into the flour with a pastry blender, or (preferably) a food processor, pulsing only until dough looks like it is comprised of little pea sized dough bits.

Second, water is used to bind the dough, but since you want to use only the minimum amount of water, it must be icy cold (water molecules change shape as they chill and give more volume than warm or room temperature water). Third, the bottom crust should be painted with egg white to keep the filling from making the crust soggy. Fourth, the pie crust must be thoroughly chilled prior to baking, and finally, the pie must be baked in a completely pre-heated, hot oven (450).

Why are these things important? For a nice crust, you want the particles of fat to burst in the flour-water paste; this bursting action is what creates flaky layers of dough. To encourage this bursting, the difference between the temperature of the dough and the oven should be as great as possible. This will shock the fat into bursting. So, the dough must be well chilled prior to baking, and the oven completely preheated. If the oven is still warming when the pie goes in, the fat will begin to melt gradually, preventing the bursting action.

If you want to try a pie crust recipe you have found elsewhere, or the one that follows, be sure you preheat your oven, chill your crust prior to baking and don't cream or over blend your shortening. If you are using CF Margarine, you should use the oleo straight from the refrigerator. Although margarine has a higher melting point than butter, it will begin to soften as it is cut into the flour, so you're best starting with it reasonably hard. If tolerated you could use a solid shortening.

Even if you follow all these guidelines, baking a GF pie crust that tastes like the real thing is no walk in the park. Good luck and keep trying. The world is still waiting for the perfect GF crust!

GF Double Crust

Many communities have Celiac support groups, and often food is brought and recipes traded at these group meetings. Susan Larson, a member of a mid-western support group tasted a pie that was brought to a recent meeting, and everyone present clamored for the recipe. Susan's mother is a wonderful pie baker, and since she missed her mom's creations Susan was thrilled to find a way to make a good crust herself. I made a few minor changed to conform to the guidelines given above.

Ingredients:

1 1/4 Cup	Rice flour
1 tsp.	Salt
2/3 Cup	Shortening, solid white or CF margarine (chilled)
1/2 Cup	Ice water
1 TBL.	Potato Flour (this time, it really is potato flour, not potato starch)

Combine water and potato flour with an electric beater or a whisk. Set aside.

Combine rice flour and salt in a bowl or food processor. Cut in shortening with a pastry blender or use short pulses of a food processor to achieve the pea consistency.

Add the potato-ice water to the rice flour mixture. If using a food processor, use short pulses and process only until the dough forms a ball. If working by hand, pour the potato water mix over the rice flour and work in with a spoon. Remove from bowl and knead gently ONLY until smooth—use as few strokes as possible.

The dough can be patted into the bottom and sides of a pie pan, or can be rolled out between sheets of wax paper that has been dusted with rice flour. Flute edges. This recipe can be used for pies that call for either a baked or unbaked crust.

For baked crust, chill and then bake in a preheated oven at 450 until brown, about 12-15 minutes.

"Graham" Cracker Crust

Health Valley makes a wonderful ersatz graham cracker called Rice Bran Crackers. They were removed from the market for a time last year, but the outcry from the GF eating public was loud and clear. They are once again available at health food stores.

Ingredients:

1 pkg.	Healthy Valley Rice Bran crackers. Blended or processed to crumbs
1/4 Cup	Sugar
1/4 Cup	CF margarine, softened
1/2 tsp.	Cinnamon (optional)

Combine all ingredients in a large mixing bowl. Mix until well blended. Place crumbs into a 9" pie pan and press into the bottom and up the sides of the pan. Bake crust at 350 for 6-8 minutes, until slightly toasted. Cool slightly before spooning in cooked pie filling.

Variations:

Flaked coconut (sulfite-free) makes a very good addition to this crust. Use 1/4 Cup pecan or almond meal to enhance a graham crust.

For banana pie, line the bottom of the crust with sliced bananas prior to filling with vanilla custard or pudding. Toss additional slices of banana with lemon juice to prevent browning, and place a border of sliced banana around the circumference of the pie.

Chocolate Pie Crust

This one is for certified chocoholics only. It cannot be used for fillings that require freezing, because the crust would be too hard to cut. If the filling requires refrigeration, remove from the refrigerator one half-hour before serving, so the crust will soften enough to cut.

Ingredients:

12 oz.	Chocolate Chips
1 TBL.	Shortening (preferably a solid white vegetable fat)
	Chopped nuts of your choice
	Flaky coconut, optional

Line an 8" or 9" pie pan with foil. Spray with vegetable spray.

Melt the chips in microwave or double boiler. Melt in shortening and then stir in nuts and coconut (if desired). Spoon the hot chocolate mixture into the pan, and spread until it covers the bottom and sides.

Chill until hardened. Remove from pan carefully, and peel off the foil. Fit crust back into the pie pan and spoon in the filling of your choice.

Meringue Crust

I always think of this as an upside down meringue pie. I usually fill the crust with a lemon meringue pie filling, but a mousse or pudding is good too. Be sure the filling is well chilled; stir it well and spoon into the shell just before serving. This crust should be light and crispy; if filled too early the shell will become soggy.

Ingredients:

4	Egg whites
1/2 tsp.	Salt
1/4 tsp.	Cream of tartar
1 Cup	Sugar
1/3 Cup	Toasted nuts, chopped fine (optional)

Preheat the oven to 200.

Beat the egg whites, salt and cream of tartar at high speed until foamy. Beat in the sugar a little at a time, until stiff peaks form.

Use a pastry bag fitted with a star tip to fill a 9" pie pan with meringue (if you don't have a pastry bag, you can use a spoon). Build up the rim of the crust 1" above the pan. Sprinkle the bottom with the chopped nuts, if desired and bake one hour until the crust sets.

Turn off the heat and leave the crust in the oven until it is completely dry. Leave it in at least two hours—if you make the crust in the evening, you can leave it in the unopened oven overnight.

Just prior to serving, fill as desired.

Hint: You can use the meringue to make little baskets that can be filled with fruit and sorbet, or fruit and pudding. These are tasty, pretty and fun to eat. To make baskets, use a parchment lined cookie sheet instead of a pie pan. Use a pastry bag to pipe circles of meringue to the desired circumference. You may want to use a cup or the bottom of a glass to draw a guideline on the paper; this will ensure that each basket is the same size.

Build up the sides by piping ropes of meringue over the round bottom and building to a height of about 2". Bake and dry as for pie crust.

Rice Crust

Another unusual crust can be made from cooked rice. It makes a nice crust for various fillings that require pre-baked crusts.

Ingredients:

2-3 Cups	Brown rice, cooked (amount depends on size of pan)
1/4 Cup	Sugar
2	Egg whites
1 tsp.	Cinnamon

Combine cooked rice with other ingredients. Press into a pie pan and bake at 350 for 10-15 minutes until it just starts to brown. Cool before filling.

Lemon Chiffon Pie

When I was a chid, my mother used to make lemon chiffon pie now and then. It wasn't much trouble; after all, it came out of a Jell-O brand box! We all loved it, and recently I began scouring the shelves of every market to find it. No luck. I called the company, to be told that while it was popular for years, it had been discontinued. I was determined to make this pie though. The following recipe is delicious and pretty darn close to the pie I recall.

Ingredients:

1	GF Graham crust, baked (see recipe above)
1	Recipe fluffy boiled white frosting (see recipe above)
1/4 Cup	Sugar
1/4 Cup	Cornstarch (use arrowroot if corn is not tolerated)

1/4 tsp.	Salt
1 Cup	Water, cold
1 Cup	Lemon juice, freshly squeezed
4	Egg yolks, lightly beaten
3 TBL.	CF Margarine

Beat egg yolks lightly and set aside.

In the top of a double boiler set over boiling water, combine sugar, cornstarch and salt.

Gradually add water and lemon juice, and mix with a wire whisk until smooth. Cook over medium heat, stirring constantly, until it thickens.

Add 1 cup of hot mixture to egg yolks and stir. Then add egg mixture back to the lemon mixture and cook over boiling water until it just starts to boil. Remove from heat and stir in margarine.

Allow filling to cool almost completely, then fold in 2-3 Tablespoons of the Fluffy Boiled Frosting to lighten the mixture. Add the rest of the meringue, folding carefully to avoid deflating.

Pour lemon/meringue mixture into the cooled crust. Refrigerate for several hours, until the filling firms up (it won't become hard). Serve cold.

NOTES

Chapter 12
Odds and Ends

What you will find here are recipes that didn't seem to fit in anywhere else—including one that isn't edible! I also have a few suggestions for lunch boxes, which is a perennial problem for most moms and dads in charge of sending food to school. Because these recipes really are odds and ends, they aren't in any particular order, ..it's a real potpourri.

Dill Pickles - by the jar

It's love or hateful these sour goodies! Sam adores pickles and Jake won't let them touch his lips. When my mother makes these, she starts with several baskets of pickling cukes and makes quarts of pickling brine. Since I never make more than a few jars at a time, she was able to cut down her recipe to one that will work for whatever number of jars you want to put up. You can even put up a single jar, but I don't advise it, as they are really good. My only change is using apple cider vinegar instead of distilled.

Ingredients for each jar:

1 TBL. (heaping)	Kosher salt
2 TBL.	Apple cider vinegar
1 TBL.	Pickling spice
1	Clove garlic, peeled
2-3	Sprigs fresh dill
	Small, crisp cucumbers (ask for pickling cucumbers)

Boiling water

Sterilize jars and lids. I run the jars through a dishwasher cycle and boil the lids in a saucepan according to the directions on the package of lids. Lids can only be used once.

To each jar, first add all the ingredients except cucumbers and water. Pack in as many cucumbers as you can, using oddly shaped cucumbers to fit the open spaces. You can slice a couple to fit in tight spots, but they will not be as crispy as the whole ones.

Bring water to a boil and pour into the filled jars. Seal with sterilized jar lids. Turn jar a few times to distribute the spices. Keep at room temperature for at least two weeks. Be patient— if you open them too early they will only be slightly pickled.

Chill the jar well before serving.

NOTE: green tomatoes can be pickled in the same way, and are delicious.

Bread and Butter Pickles

My mother rarely made these pickles, which are truly wonderful. My grandmother made them, and everyone in my family (except Jake!) loves them too. As is usual for my Bubby's recipes, there are no real measurements. You'll have to wing it as I always do! This recipe is forgiving however, and very tasty. Again, the only modification I have made from the original recipe is to use apple cider vinegar. To estimate the right amount of syrup needed, determine the (approximate) number of jars your ingredients will fill. Then calculate everything on that number. Remember, when filled with cukes your quart jar won't hold a quart of water! I usually don't make these pickles in quart sized jars—for some reason the pint sized jar seems better for B&B pickles.

Ingredients:

1 Part	Apple Cider Vinegar
2 Parts	Sugar
	Salt
	Turmeric (use at least a teaspoon per jar)
	Pickling spice (use at least a Tablespoon per jar)
	Water: use 1 Cup water for each cup of vinegar

Boil the above ingredients together. Once they have come to a good strong boil, add: Sweet red peppers, chopped Cauliflower, broken into small flowerets, Sliced onion (or whole pearl onions), and Cucumbers sliced into 1/4-1/2" thick rounds.

Return the pot to a boil and cook for about 2 minutes.

Pack the cucumbers into sterilized jars, then cover with syrup mixture. Be sure a few vegetables go into each jar.

Seal as per package directions for lids. Keep at room temperature for one week to 10 days. Chill a jar and enjoy.

Ketchup

Yes, I said Ketchup. My son would eat ketchup on everything, if allowed. You can use prepared ketchup, but be sure to call the company that makes your favorite brand—sometimes the natural flavorings are not GF. If you cannot find one that is, or you just want to try something new, here's a pretty easy way to make it yourself.

Ingredients:

12	Plum tomatoes, chopped
1	Onion, chopped very fine

2	Cloves garlic, minced fine
1 1/4 tsp.	Salt
1	Red pepper, chopped very fine
1 1/2 tsp.	Celery seeds
1/2 tsp.	Cayenne pepper
1/2 tsp.	Cinnamon
2 TBL.	Sugar (can use other sweetener)
1/2 Cup	Apple cider vinegar

Boil tomatoes, onions, garlic, salt, and pepper for about 30 minutes, until reduced to a sauce.

Strain through a sieve and discard the solids.

Place spices in a *bouquet garni* or wrap in cheesecloth, closing with string or a twist-tie. Place in the sauce, and stir in the sugar. Simmer slowly, stirring often, for 25-30 minutes.

Add the vinegar and remove the spices. Simmer on low heat for another 10-12 minutes.

Cool and pour into a sterilized jar or jars (this recipe makes approximately one quart of ketchup).

Seal as directed on jar/lid packages for later use. Since ketchup only lasts for a month after opening, you will probably want to pack it in small jars. Sealed jars will last for six months.

"Mock Cheese Sauce"

*This food is similar to the processed cheese spreads that come in tubes or bottles. Not exactly camembert, but not too bad poured on a burger. You could also use this for mock macaroni and cheese (Chapter 6) instead of the white sauce base or added to it. It certainly **looks** like Cheese sauce, although the taste is quite distinctive.*

In a blender combine:

15 oz.	Canned white beans, carefully rinsed
1/2 Cup	Bottled pimentos, drained well
2-3 TBL.	Fresh lemon juice
3 TBL.	Tahini
1/2 tsp.	Onion powder
1/4 tsp.	Garlic powder
1/2 tsp.	Mustard
1 tsp.	Turmeric (start with 1/2 tsp. and add until you reached desired color)
	Salt, to taste

Refrigerate in covered container and use within a week.

Mock Cheese

This is a really good cheese-type food it is the third and last of Beth Crowell's recipes that I will share with you. If you want more, you'll have to get her book yourself!

Ingredients:

1 1/2 Cups	Water
5 TBL.	Agar Flakes (found in health food or Asian stores)
3/4 Cup	Cashew pieces, cashew butter or tahini (or a combination)
1 1/4 tsp.	Salt
2 tsp.	Onion powder
1/4 tsp.	Garlic powder
1/4 Cup	Pimentos

2 1/2 TBL.   Lemon Juice (Must be freshly squeezed!)

Combine water and agar in a small saucepan. Cook over medium heat, stirring frequently until boiling. Reduce heat and simmer for 5 minutes, stirring occasionally.

Combine other ingredients in a blender or food processor. Add the hot agar and water, and blend on high for 1-2 minutes, stopping to stir when necessary.

Pour into a mold, or in an 8" x 8" pan lined with plastic wrap. Chill until firm.

This cheese is firm enough to be grated, but freezing it for a time will make grating even easier.

For softer cheese, reduce the amount of agar to 4 Tablespoons. For a spread reduce it to 3 Tablespoons and for a dip use only 1 1/2 Tablespoons agar.

You can flavor the cheese anyway you like. Beth suggests: add 2 Tablespoons dill or 1 1/2 Tablespoons caraway seeds, or 1 Tablespoon or more finely diced onion or scallions. Peppers (diced), black olives, green olives and vegetable flakes also make good additions.

Fresh Salsa

This is an easy salsa to put together as a recipe ingredient, or just for dipping some tortilla chips. Be sure to find fresh cilantro...it makes a big difference in the taste. If you don't find cilantro easily, try growing it from seeds. They are easy to grow even in little indoor herb pots. The seeds can be ground and used too-the seed form of the plant is called coriander, and has a completely different flavor and character from the leaves. If the seeds fall on the dirt, you'll have a new crop of cilantro again in a few months. I do not give measurements because you can vary the proportion of the ingredients to taste. It also depends on how much salsa you want to make.

Ingredients:

Chopped tomatoes, seeded

Chopped onion

Jalapeno, roasted, peeled and seeded (omit if you don't want it spicy)

Cilantro, chopped

Apple cider vinegar

Cayenne pepper (optional—for heat)

Salt

Blend all the ingredients except vinegar. Use the vinegar to achieve the right consistency. For a thicker dip, puree a can of (drained and rinsed) black beans and add to the salsa.

Egg-free Egg Salad

If you're an egg salad lover, this high protein sandwich filler will please you. It can be eaten with impunity, especially if you choose a light mayo. I have used the ingredients I always used for my "real" egg salad—feel free to substitute those your family likes.

Ingredients:

1 pkg.	Silken tofu, firm (light versions are fine)
2 TBL.	Light mayonnaise (check ingredients carefully)
1 TBL.	Sweet pickle relish (or chopped Bread & Butter pickles)
1/2 tsp.	Salt
1/2 tsp.	Celery seed
1/2 tsp.	Dry prepared mustard (for color)

Crumble tofu in a small bowl until it looks like chopped egg white. Add other ingredients and mix thoroughly to distribute the color. Cover with plastic wrap and chill.

Granola

Granola is a delicious snack and when you add a few pieces of chocolate and nuts you have Gorp, a must for overnight camping trips (or long hikes). Granola is also delicious when added to muffins, or baked into cookies. For example, an Oatmeal cookie recipe could be converted to GF by exchanging the flour, and using granola in place of the oatmeal (remember to reduce the sugar as the granola is sweet). It is rich to eat as a breakfast cereal, but is delicious when a few spoonfuls are added to a plain bowl office or corn cereal. Add whatever you have and your child likes.

Ingredients:

3 Cups	Puffed rice
3 Cups	GF Corn flakes, crushed (if tolerated)
1 Cup	Perky's Nutty Rice cereal
1 Cup	Almonds (any nuts that are tolerated can be used, alone or in combination)
1 Cup	Sunflower seeds
1 Cup	Soy nuts (if tolerated)
1/3 Cup	Honey or GF Rice Syrup
1/3 Cup	Canola or other vegetable oil
1 Cup	Raisins
1 Cup	Dried fruit (I always add dried cherries—see Appendix I)
1 Cup	Dried coconut (unsulfited)

Preheat oven to 225. Coat a large roaster pan with vegetable spray. Add all nuts, seeds, and cereals.

In a saucepan, combine oil and honey and bring to a boil, stirring constantly. Pour this mixture over the granola ingredients and stir very well to coat all ingredients.

Bake for 2 hours. Add dried fruits and raisins after baking, and stir well. Let granola come to room temperature, then store in airtight containers.

Vanilla Pudding Mix

Vance's DariFree™ is a wonderful milk substitute that has a potato base. It works particularly well for puddings and cream soups you want to thicken. It has a very pleasant taste, and works well in this pudding mix recipe. Having some of this on hand will allow you to whip up pudding or a pie filling in no time.

Ingredients:

3 Cups	Vance's DariFree™
1 1/2 Cups	Sugar
1 1/2 Cups	Arrowroot starch or tapioca starch
1 1/2 tsp.	Salt
4 tsp.	Xanthan gum
2 Packets	Unflavored gelatin

Combine ingredients thoroughly. Divide into 1 Cup batches and store in airtight containers.

To Make Pudding:

1 Batch	Pudding mix
3/4 Cup	Milk substitute (liquid Darifree or soy milk work best)

1 Cup	Water (reduce to 3/4 Cup for a thicker pudding)
1	Egg, beaten (or egg substitute)
1 tsp.	Vanilla
1 TBL.	CF margarine

Empty mix into a 1-2 quart saucepan. Over low heat, add milk and water slowly. Whisk until smooth.

Raise heat to medium, and cook, stirring constantly until the pudding thickens and small bubbles begin to form around the edges of the pan. Cook 2-3 minutes longer, stirring constantly to prevent scorching. Remove from heat.

Stir vanilla into beaten egg, and then whisk 1/2 cup hot pudding into the egg mixture.

Return pudding-egg mixture to the saucepan. Add CF margarine and stir well.

If lumps form, strain as you pour the pudding into serving cups or ramekins. To prevent a pudding skin from forming, cover with plastic wrap and chill well. When you remove the plastic the skin will come off too. If you like the skin, chill uncovered.

Chocolate Pudding Mix

Similar to the recipe for vanilla pudding, this recipe contains no egg.

Ingredients:

2 1/4 Cups	Vance's DariFree™
1 Cup	Sugar
1/2 Cup	Arrowroot starch or tapioca starch
2/3 Cup	Unsweetened cocoa, sifted

1/4 tsp.	Salt
4 tsp.	Xanthan gum
2 Packets	Unflavored gelatin

Combine well and divide into four batches. Store each in airtight container.

To Make Pudding:

1 Batch	Pudding mix
3/4 Cup	Water
1 Cup	Milk (use DariFree or Soy milk)
1 TBL.	CF margarine
1/2 tsp.	Vanilla

Empty mix into 1 or 2 quart saucepan. Gradually stir in water and milk and bring to a boil over medium heat, stirring constantly to prevent scorching. Reduce heat and simmer for 2 more minutes, stirring constantly.

Remove from heat and stir in butter and vanilla. Strain into serving cups, cover with plastic (as described for Vanilla pudding) and chill.

Waldorf Salad

If your child cannot tolerate apples, substitute firm pears. Some children may find this too tart, but others will like it. It was a favorite in my family. Tiny GF marshmallows can be added if desired. It is very easy to make and is great for a picnic. The amounts are up to you...use as much as necessary to feed your crew.

Ingredients:

Apples, chopped

Celery, chopped

White raisin

Walnuts, chopped (if tolerated)

Dressing: 2-3 Tablespoons GF mayonnaise thinned with pear, orange or pineapple juice.

Combine ingredients, top with dressing and chill before serving.

Pearsauce

When Sam was first eating solid food, I tried to make many things from scratch, including zwieback crackers and other baby foods. I nearly always made applesauce, since it tasted so much better than store bought, and had a lot less sugar. It is delicious on its own or served with potato pancakes or pork chops. Because so many children should avoid apples, I make this sauce instead. It can be used in any recipe that calls for applesauce. Many people use applesauce in place of oil or margarine when they bake. This sauce will work too, but with GF flours it is not always a reliable substitute. This recipe makes only about two cups, but could certainly be doubled.

Ingredients:

2 lb.	Pears (approx. 6 large)
1/4 Cup	Water (approximately)
2 TBL.	Sugar (if fruit is sweet, decrease or eliminate sweetener)
1/2 tsp.	Cinnamon (optional)
1/4 tsp.	Nutmeg (freshly grated is best)

Use a variety of pear that your family enjoys. Peel and chop the fruit—the smaller the pieces the more quickly the sauce will cook.

Place the fruit in a saucepan with 2-3 Tablespoons water. On medium heat cook, stirring, until the fruit begins to bubble. Lower the heat and cook, stirring often. When the fruit needs more liquid to cook, add water a few Tablespoons at a time (up to 1/4 - 1/3 Cups total).

Add a few Tablespoons sugar if the fruit is tart. If not, you may not need to add any sugar at all.

Cinnamon sprinkled in adds nice flavor. For variety, some diced, dried fruit (e.g. apricots or cherries) can be added to the pears. This addition adds sweetness so if you do add dried fruit you won't want to use much sugar.

The fruit is done when the largest pieces have cooked down to small ones, and the smallest have disappeared into the sauce.

The sauce is tasty in this chunky style, but most children prefer it smooth. Also, if you plan to bake with it you will want to get rid of the chunks. To do so, transfer the sauce to a blender or food processor (I always use a Braun®Multipractic, a hand-held blender that can be immersed directly into the pot. This gadget is great for pureeing soups too).

Confectioner's Sugar

Since confectioner's sugar always contains cornstarch, you will need to make your own if you want to have it on hand and your child can't tolerate corn. It isn't hard to do, but it does require a food processor. A blender simply isn't powerful enough. I suggest making 5 lb. at a time, and burying a split vanilla bean in one of the containers for vanilla scented confectioner's sugar.

Ingredients:

5 lb.   Sugar

Fit the bowl of your food processor with the steel blade and process until the sugar is the proper consistency.

Corn-Free Marshmallows

Marshmallows are generally made with confectioner's sugar, which contains cornstarch. Another listed ingredient will either be modified food starch or more cornstarch. Either way, if your child cannot tolerate corn then he or she cannot eat them. Fortunately, they are not hard to make, and either arrowroot powder or tapioca starch can be substituted for the corn. To make this recipe, you will first need to make your own confectioner's sugar (see recipe above).

Ingredients:

1/4 Cup	Arrowroot or tapioca starch
1/3 Cup	Corn-free confectioner's sugar
1 envelope	Unflavored gelatin
1/3 Cup	Water
2/3 Cup	Sugar (granulated)
1/4 Cup	100% Pure Vegetable Glycerine
OR	
1/2 Cup	GF Brown rice syrup
2 tsp.	Vanilla flavoring (optional if you use Vanilla sugar)
Pinch	Salt

Sift the starch and confectioner's sugar into a bowl. Set aside.

Spray an 8"x 8" square pan and sprinkle in 1 Tablespoon of the starch and sugar mixture. Tilt to cover bottom and sides of pan. Leave any excess in the pan.

Sprinkle the gelatin into the water in a small pan and let soften for 5 minutes. Add the granulated sugar and stir over low heat until the gelatin and sugar dissolve. In the bowl of an electric mixer, combine the gelatin mixture, syrup, salt and vanilla and beat for 15 minutes on high speed, until peaks form.

Spread this mixture into the prepared pan and smooth the top. Allow to set at room temperature, about 2 hours. With a wet knife, cut mixture into quarters and loosen sides. Sprinkle remaining starch/sugar mixture onto a cookie sheet and invert the marshmallow blocks. Cut each quarter into nine pieces and roll each one in starch and sugar. Place the marshmallows on a rack covered with paper towels and allow them to stand overnight to dry the surface. Store airtight for up to a month.

TIP: For Marshmallow cream, use immediately after beating.

Hot Chocolate Mix

No reason that making hot cocoa should be any harder than opening one of those premixed packets!

Ingredients:

4 Cups	DariFree, Better Than Milk or Rice Moo
3/4 Cup	Unsweetened cocoa powder
1 1/2 Cups	Sugar (preferably vanilla sugar)
1/8 tsp.	Salt

Combine all ingredients and store in an airtight container. To use, place 3 Tablespoons mix in a cup. Add a small amount of boiling water and stir to dissolve mix. Fill cup with boiling water.

Lollipops

Surprisingly, lollipops aren't very hard to make at home. This is not something I make often, and hardly suggest that they be a regular part of the diet! But around Valentine's Day, Halloween and Christmas, school parties abound and treats are everywhere. If you make these, your child will also have a treat. True, they are full of demon sugar, but at least you can avoid the artificial flavorings and colors. To make lollipops you will need candy molds—any store that sells candy-making supplies will have them. Be sure to buy molds that are intended for hard candy and not chocolate (chocolate molds will melt when you pour in 310 candy) Many candy thermometers are not suitable for small batches of candy. If you can find one that will give an accurate reading in a low volume, great. If not, use the old fashioned method given at the end of the recipes.

Butterscotch Lollipops

Ingredients:

1 Cup	Light brown sugar
1/4 Cup	CF margarine
2 TBL.	Light corn syrup, or rice syrup
1 TBL.	Water
1 TBL.	Cider vinegar

Equipment:

Candy molds

Lollipop sticks

Cellophane lollipop bags

Curling ribbon or twist ties

Accurate Candy thermometer OR Large bowl filled with icy cold water

Spray molds with vegetable spray and place a stick in the indentation of each one. Set oiled molds in a convenient place, near but not too near the stovetop. Make sure the molds are on a completely flat surface.

Place all ingredients in the top of a double boiler and cook over medium heat. Stir only until the syrup is clear and boiling. Cover the pot and let it cook for 3 minutes.

Uncover the pot and insert the thermometer. Boil vigorously until it measures 260. Reduce the heat and boil more gently until the thermometer reads at least 300.

Remove from heat, stir to eliminate bubbles and pour into molds. Wait 15 minutes and lift lollipops out of mold by holding the stick.

Maple Lollipops

Ingredients:

    1 1/2 Cups   Pure Maple Syrup

Same equipment and directions as for butterscotch pops.

If you do not have a candy thermometer, follow candy-making directions below.

Old fashioned Candy-Making Technique

This is much less intimidating than it seems. You can be successful, even on the first try. Be sure that you have sprayed the molds with vegetable spray (not too much) and put the sticks in place. They should be on a flat surface. If your countertop cannot take intense heat, place the molds on a wooden board or on a few layers of paper toweling.

  1.   Prepare icy water and place very near the stovetop (but away from the heat).

2. Place all ingredients in a 2 quart sauce pan over medium heat. Stir with a wooden spoon to mix, then cook without stirring for 5 minutes.

3. After 5 minutes, remove a teaspoon of the syrup and drop it into the icy water. Reach into the water and see if you can grab it into a **soft ball**. It should be pliable and easy to form. If it isn't at this soft ball stage, keep testing every 30 seconds to be sure it reaches this stage. If it does not reach soft ball within a few minutes, increase the heat.

4. Cook for a few more minutes then test again. The next stage is firm ball, in which you can gather it into a ball, but the ball hardens quickly and is more difficult to squeeze out of shape.

5. Soon after reaching this stage it will reach hard ball stage—it will form a ball but you cannot squeeze it out of shape.

6. Now you should be testing every minute or so, until it reaches the soft crack stage, in which the syrup forms long threads when it falls into the water. The strands will be soft, first bending and then breaking.

7. Once it's reached soft crack, check again right away, because it will quickly go to the hard crack stage. It must reach hard crack to be made into lollipops. At this stage the strands are very crisp and crunchy.

8. At hard crack, remove the pan from the heat. Stir briefly to remove as many bubbles as possible.

9. Pour the syrup into prepared molds.

10. Wait 15 minutes and then unmold candies by lifting the stick out of the mold.

Hint: I keep a large pyrex measuring cup nearby (coated with vegetable spray). I like to pour the hot syrup into the cup, which makes pouring into the molds accurately a lot easier. For clean-up, use very hot water to melt off the syrup left in the saucepan and cup.

Bert's Nut Candy

My mother used to bring this candy when she visited, but Serge liked it so much that I had to start making it myself. I knew it only had two ingredients, but I had my mom "walk me through it" over the phone the first time I made it. Bags of this candy find their way into everyone's holiday package, and you can make a big batch much more quickly than you can make a large quantity of cookies. When time gets pressured, I always end up using more candy than anything else for edible gifts. Parchment paper is essential.

Ingredients:

Nuts	Amount and type of your choice
Sugar	Determined by the amount of nuts you are using

Place a bath towel on a table or counter surface. Cover this with parchment paper.

Pour nuts into a large, heavy skillet, preferably with a non-stick coating. You can have more than just a flat layer of nuts, but the more nuts you have the harder it will be to make the recipe.

You are better off making more batches than crowding lots of nuts in the pan.

I generally use a combination of pecans, walnuts and cashews. Any nut will work.

Place the pan of nuts on the stove and add sugar. To determine how much is enough you will have to eyeball it and guess! You want a thick layer of sugar to cover the nuts, but the nuts will still peek through. For 2 10 oz bags of nuts I use about 3 Cups of sugar.

Turn the heat to medium high. After a very few minutes, begin to stir. The sugar will begin to melt slowly, and at first it will look like a real mess. The sugar will melt into hard, light brown lumps. Soon these lumps will start sticking to the nuts, but they will still be distinct lumps and the whole thing will look pretty awful.

Keep stirring at all times! Within 10 minutes, the lumps will begin to melt into the nuts. Before you know it, they will have been replaced by a beautiful, evenly colored brown caramel.

Keep stirring at all times! If you don't this will burn and once burned they are beyond redemption.

When all sugar has caramelized, make sure all nuts are coated. You will have more caramel than nuts...don't worry about it. Next, quickly pour the nuts on to the parchment. Use a wooden spoon to help the nuts out of the pan and to spread them out as much as possible. Let any extra caramel pour over the nuts.

Be careful! Hot sugar will make a terrible burn if you get it on your hands. Let the candy cool completely, then break it into pieces and store airtight. Candy freezes well. When packaged attractively, this candy makes fabulous gifts.

Nuant

Karyn Seroussi calls this treat either Nuant or 'Jewish Nut Candy." I had never heard of it until she gave me the recipe. She uses macadamia nuts, because her son doesn't tolerate most nuts. These are delicious, but very expensive. If your child can eat other nuts, you might want to try something else. You can also use a very crispy cereal instead, such as Perky's Nutty Rice if no nuts are tolerated. These couldn't be easier.

Ingredients:

1 Cup	Honey
1 TBL.	Lemon juice
3 1/2 Cups	Nuts, chopped (or crunchy GF cereal)

Bring honey and lemon juice to a boil, stirring constantly with a wooden spoon. Add nuts and keep stirring until the mixture is thick and golden, about 2 minutes.

Pour into a greased pan and pat with a wooden spoon to a 3/4" thickness. Cool and cut into 1" squares.

Chocolate Syrup

Although Nestles and other brands of chocolate milk makers are GF, they are usually filled with preservatives and other additives. Here is a recipe that the Feingold Association recommends for making chocolate milk.

Ingredients:

1/4 Cup	Water
1/2 Cup	Sugar
1/4 Cup	Cocoa
Dash	Salt

Boil water and add the sugar and cocoa to the pan. Heat, stirring until dissolved, then remove from heat.

Store in a glass jar and refrigerate. To make chocolate milk add 2-3 Tablespoons syrup to 8 oz. of the CF milk of your choice.

Play Clay

Most children like play clay, but the most commonly used brands actually contain wheat! At many daycare centers and preschools, play clay is made on site, reducing the cost and giving the children a fun activity. Although some teachers follow the recipe on the Arm and Hammer® baking soda box, most use flour based recipes. There are several ways to make this clay and you should try one, especially if your child is a clay eater (as many children are). In fact, there is even an edible version you can try if your child insists on nibbling on his or her artistic creations. If you use an edible version, do not use food coloring (or use natural pigments such as beet juice). Even if your child does not deliberately eat clay, it does tend to adhere to little hands and get under nails, and could easily be transferred to the mouth inadvertently.

Ingredients:

1/2 Cup	Rice flour
1/2 Cup	Corn starch
1 tsp.	Salt
2 tsp.	Cream of tartar
1 Cup	Water
1 tsp.	Cooking oil
	Food coloring

Combine all ingredients in a pot and cook over low heat until it forms a ball. When cool enough to touch, pat gently until smooth. When completely cool, store in an airtight container.

Edible Play Clay

This clay is good for sculpting or playing with, and it can be eaten. It doesn't dry out if stored properly.

Ingredients:

1/3 Cup	CF margarine

1/2 tsp.	Salt
1/3 Cup	Light corn syrup
1 tsp.	Vanilla flavoring (GF)
1 lb.	GF Confectioner's sugar

Mix the first four ingredients with a strong electric mixer. When well combined, add the powdered sugar and mix. Knead the dough until smooth, divide into desired portions and color each with natural food colors. Store in airtight containers (zipper-type plastic bags work well) and place in the refrigerator to prevent spoiling.

Appendix I
Mail Order Sources

If prepared by a good cook, home-made foods are nearly always better than store bought food or food made from a mix. But not everyone has time to cook and bake daily. And not everyone enjoys doing it. Even if you do like to bake, you may simply run out of time, dealing with children, work schedules and, well, life. Fortunately for us there are several companies out there who provide excellent "shortcuts." Some are available in health food stores, but many can only be found through mail order sources. The companies which have web sites are listed with an asterisk (*), and their URLs are given. There are probably hundreds of other good mail order companies out there, but this list contains my current favorites.

Many of these companies also carry very hard to find ingredients and equipment that will be essential if you plan to do some or all of your cooking and baking from scratch. You should be sure to get catalogues from as many of these companies as possible, or keep an eye on their web sites.

Allergy Resources: This company offers hundreds of hard-to-find products, such as snacks, cookies, dried fruits, unusual nut butters, pastas, sweeteners (including both 100% pure vegetable Glycerin and Stevia), baking mixes, MCT oil, flours and bean fibers and unusual starches (e.g. Kuzu and Taro). This company sells all the "gluten substitutes" commonly used in baking (Xanthan gum, guar gum and methycellulose). They carry vitamins, minerals, amino acids and herbs. The catalog includes various cosmetic items made without any scents or dyes. If you only get one catalog, this may be the most complete one around. Read all the ingredients on foods in this catalog—many are GF/CF but not all. **1-303-438-0600**

*American Spoon Foods: This Michigan company sells wonderful sauces, salad dressings, jams, "spoon fruit" and tart dried cherries that are better than any others. Their fruit butters and spoon fruits are jams made from lovely fruits, and sweetened only by concentrated juices. Their dried fruits and nuts make wonderful additions to many different types of recipes. A great source. **1-800-222-5886**. www.spoon.com

*Authentic Foods: This California company advertises that they offer GF mixes "with a difference!" Their bread, cookie, cake and other mixes are made with a social bean flour. This flour is a combination of garbanzo (chickpea) and lava beans. Their chocolate cake mix is terrific. You can also buy the flours and make your own. **1-213-934-0424**. www.authenticfoods.com

Celia Cooks: This mail order company specializes in GF "gourmet and convenience foods" which are packaged as easy-to-prepare dinners. For more information call **1-800-717-0005** or send email to: celiacooks@aol.com.

David's Goodbatter: This company's bread, cake and cookie mixes are generally available at health food stores, but they do have mail order if you can't find them. Their chocolate cake mix is excellent. Read the labels carefully; not all the products are gluten-free. **1-717-872-0652**.

*Dietary Specialties: This company carries many baking ingredients, mixes, snacks, pastas etc. They even carry condiments, such as pickles, mustard and various sauces. **1-716-263-2787**. www.dietspec.com

*Ener-G Foods: Call for a complete list of products. They sell xanthan gum (essential for giving gluten-free baked products the proper texture). The "GF Gourmet Blend" is the Hagman GF flour mix Ener-g sells this in one pound pouches or 5 pound bags. These products are available at most health food stores, or you can order via phone or mail. **1-800-331-5222**. www.ener-g.com

*G! FOODS: G! Foods is a San Francisco based mail-order supplier of gluten-free cookies and snacks. They use organic grains and "healthy hen" eggs in their products. **1-415-255-2139**. www.g-foods.com

The Gluten-Free Cookie Jar: This company, located in Trevose, PA, sells many pre-baked cookies, muffins, breads, cakes and more. They sell a small selection of mixes, but their main appeal is the fact that they have such a wide selection of prepared foods. **1-215-355-9403**

Gluten-Free Delights: This company sells many delicious products, but if your family is pining for English muffins or donuts, this is the place to call. They also make excellent cookies. **1-319-266-7167**.

*The Gluten-Free Pantry: The GF Pantry is known for its excellent mixes for breads, cookies and pancakes, cakes, bagels, baking ingredients and much, much more. Some mixes are sold in health food stores, but the full line is available only through mail order. They also carry bread machines and various other non-food items that make this diet easier to manage. Read ingredients carefully, however, as not all mixes are dairy-free. Orders are accepted via phone **1-203-633-3826**, fax or Internet; www.glutenfree.com

*Indian Harvest: Indian Harvest calls itself "the ultimate in rice, grain and bean catalogue" and they may not be exaggerating. Though not all their products are GF, many are. They have unusual pilaf blends and an excellent assortment of beans and legumes. Unusual bean, lentil and corn varieties too. www.indianharvest.com

*King Arthur Flour: Although this company's main products are wheat based, they also carry tapioca flour, white rice flour, potato starch flour, xanthan gum. They have many interesting "add- ins" for baking, and hard to find baking utensils (e.g. they carry cracker making tools). They are a good source of dehydrated egg whites and of meringue powder that does not contain additives. **1-800-827-6836**. www.kingarrthurflouncom

*Kinnikinnick Foods: This Canadian company has everything you might need, including ingredients, mixes, condiments, baked foods. Kinnikinnick is one of the few places that stocks rice flakes, which can be used in place of oatmeal in cereal, cookies and as a binding in meat loaf and other meats. Now has a casein-free line. **1-403-433-4023**. www.kinnikinnick.com

*Jowar Foods: If you can't find jowar (sorghum) flour locally, this is the place! They sell the flour and various mixes and products made from it. **1-800-363-9070**. www.jowar.com

KCJ Vanilla Company: While they don't specialize in GF or CF products, this company carries wonderful natural flavorings, citrus oils, hard to find black walnuts, and of course, vanilla and vanilla beans. If you don't want to make "vanilla sugar," their vanilla powder is an excellent substitute for extract. It contains no alcohol or sugar and can be added to any recipes that call for vanilla extract. Write to the company at PO Box 126, Norwood, PA 19074.

*Lundberg Family Farms: Most of this company's products are available at groceries and health food stores. They are very helpful, however, if you need advice on a product or other information. It was by sending them email that I obtained the recipe for Riz Cous. http://www.lundberg.com

*Omega Nutrition: This company sells everything from vitamins to nut flours. They sell some hard to find items, such as hazelnut flour and pumpkin seed spread, and are a source for natural, unprocessed coconut oil products. Omega's catalogue is also full of useful information about foods and nutrition. **1-800-661-3529**. www.omegaflo.com

The Really Great Food Co.: This company carries a selection of pancake, gingerbread, cornbread, pizza crust mixes, and more. Their pizza crust mix is very simple and makes a very good GF, yeast- free crust. I have used this (mix to make small flat breads and crackers. **1-516-593-5587**

*Miss Roben's: Miss Roben's offers excellent bread, cake, muffin, pie crust and other mixes. A really good company with very good products. **1-800-891-0083**. www.missroben.com

*Very Special Foods: This company carries the most unusual food items; if you are seeking foods that your child has never eaten for a strict elimination diet, this is the place to start. In addition to foods and flours made from water chestnuts, lotus roots, white sweet potatoes and others, the company has imitation nut butters which are made with no nuts at all (they are made from cassava, malaria, yams etc.). Unusual nut butters are available, made from pecans, pumpkin seeds, brazil nuts, macadamias, sunflower and hazelnuts. They are quite good. If requested, you can receive an "Open Letter to Parents of Autistic Children" with your catalog. **1-703-644-0991**. www.specialfoods.com

Sunnyland Farms, Inc.: This Georgia company has been selling nuts and fruits for 49 years. They are a terrific resource, because they sell quality nuts in bulk. Their prices for "home boxes" of pecans, walnuts, cashews, macadamia nuts and many others cannot be beat. A terrific company. Call for a copy of their catalogue. **1-800-999-2488**

***Tamarind Tree:** Tamarind Tree sells Indian vegetarian dinners. Indian cuisine uses many high fiber, high protein beans, mixed with rice and wonderful spices. These frozen dinners are quick to prepare and very tasty. They also sell crispy pappadams, an indian fried lentil bread which is more like a chip or very crispy cracker than a bread. You may think your children won't eat Indian food, but you could be surprised; my son loves it. Some of these dinners are available at health food stores or even supermarkets. **1-800-HFC-TREE** www.tamtree.com

Walnut Acres: Walnut Acres is a wonderful source of organic grains, fruits and other products. Most of their foods are not GF, so you must take care when ordering. But their catalog gives a complete ingredient listings. They have delicious rice blends, absolutely delicious peanut butter, nuts, fruit leathers and jams. Recently, this 51 year old company added a new line of nut and seed butters including: dark roast almond butter, roasted cashew butter, roasted hazelnut butter and roasted sunflower butter. www.walnutacres.com

Appendix II
Dairy Substitutes

All the milk substitutes listed are fortified with calcium and vitamin D. Some have additional nutrients added. Check the labels. You many want to supplement with additional calcium and vitamin D. Many of the products come in non-fat versions - read the labels carefully.

Better Than Milk?®

This tofu beverage is both lactose and casein-free (unlike some tofu-based products). It is available in 1lb. canisters (powdered) or in 32 oz. cartons (liquid). It tastes quite good, and can be used in bread and other recipes that call for dry milk. Made by Sovex Foods (1-800-227- 2320), it can typically be found in health food stores. Note: This product comes in two forms. Do not buy European Style, because it contains casein. The canisters are clearly marked as either Caseinate-Free or European Style.

EdenBlend

This drink is easily found in grocery and health food stores, and comes in 32 oz. cartons. It contains water, brown rice, soybeans, kombu (seaweed), carageenan, sea salt and calcium carbonate. Some people think it is less bean tasting than straight soy milk. It looks less appealing than other milk substitutes, as it is brownish in color. Another variety sold by Eden Foods is called **EdenRice**. They are similar, but EdenRice is sweetened with rice syrup that uses barley enzymes in processing. Edenblend is a safer choice.

Ener-G Nutquik

Nutquik consists of finely chopped blanched almonds. It is reconstituted by adding water, blending, straining and repeating the process. It starts out very thick, but eventually is milk-like in thickness. This is time-consuming, however, and the resulting liquid can be grainy. It tastes good, but you may want to use it for cooking and baking only. For drinking, there are other drink mixes which reconstitute more easily or come in liquid form. If you need almond meal or flour, Nutquik can be ground in a food processor and will work very well in most recipes. 1-800-331-5222.

Harmony Farms

This is a relative newcomer in the field of gluten/casein-free non-dairy beverages. It is very similar to Rice Dream, but is generally less expensive. I found it extremely thin and watery, but my son did eat it on cereal without complaint. A fussier child may not be happy with this substitute.

Pacific Ultra

This beverage does not, like many others, have gluten hidden in the brown rice syrup. Pacific Ultra is soy based, and also contains lactobacillus acidophilus and L. bifidus. These two ingredients are also found in the company's rice beverage, Pacific Rice. I know of no other beverage with these two 'good' bacteria. The rice drink is also casein and gluten-free, but many think it is not as tasty as the companies Pacific Ultra.

Rice Dream

Rice Dream is carried in most grocery and health food stores. It contains minute amounts of gluten from the rice syrup, but many celiacs and individuals with autism drink the plain version with impunity. The taste is pleasant enough, but it is very thin. My children don't seem to mind this but I only buy this product if no other is available. Imagine Puddings, made by the same company, are now gluten-free and very good.

RiceMoo

RiceMoo is another powdered beverage made by Sovex Foods. It also comes in a 1 lb. canister, works well in cooking and baking, and tastes good.

SoyGood

BestLife makes a soy-based beverage called SoyGood. It is casein and gluten-free. It tastes quite a bit like milk, and can be mail ordered. **1-800-407-7238**.

Vance's DariFree™

This potato-based drink tastes good and looks like milk. It has no cholesterol, lactose, soy, rice, corn, oils or MSG. It is also excellent for baking and cooking and is my personal favorite. If made with less water, it can be used as a coffee creamer. It comes in 7oz packets that yield 2 quarts each, or in 5 lb. jars (which yield 230 quarts). Some health food stores carry Darifree™, but most people will need to order it from A & A Amazing Foods, Inc. **1-800-497-4834**, or from the Autism Network for Dietary Intervention, **1-800-535-4807**.

WestSoy Plus

This drink is very good, although I prefer a product that comes in a powder so I can bake with it more easily. The color is a little on the yellow side, but looks appetizing. It is thick and very tasty, although the fat-free version is a little on the thin side. If soy is tolerated however, this is one of the better tasting drinks. It is available in most grocery and health food stores.

White Wave Silk Milk, RiceSilk and Yogurts

The White Wave Company makes good tasting fruit yogurts from soy—all of the flavors are a big hit at our house. When I saw they had a new drink out I tried it immediately. Silk Milk is an excellent soy drink, thick and tasty. It comes in quart and half gallon containers and can be found in the refrigerator section of most markets or health food stores. Both the plain and chocolate versions are excellent. For people who cannot drink soy, White Wave now makes a soy-free RiceSilk that is rice based. It too is very good. The only problem with these products is that they are quite expensive. When buying the yogurt beware of one thing: the plain yogurt is not gluten-free, although the fruit flavors are.

Appendix III
Frequently Asked Questions by Karyn A. Seroussi

(reprinted with permission of author)

Q: I don't think my child has allergies, or that allergies could cause autism. Why should I try removing foods from his diet?

A: Although parents have been reporting a connection between autism and diet for decades, there is now a growing body of research that shows that certain foods seem to be affecting the developing brains of some children and causing autistic behaviors. This is not because of allergies, but because many of these children are unable to properly break down certain proteins.

Q: What happens when they get these proteins?

A: Researchers in England, Norway, and at the University of Florida had previously found peptides (breakdown products of proteins) with opiate activity in the urine of a high percentage of autistic children. Opiates are drugs, like morphine, which affect brain function.

Q: Which proteins are causing this problem?

A: The two main offenders seem to be gluten (the protein in wheat, oats, rye and barley) and casein (milk protein).

Q: But milk and wheat are the only two foods my child will eat. His diet is completely comprised of milk, cheese, cereal, pasta, and bread. If I take these away, I'm afraid he'll starve.

A: There may be a good reason your child "self-limits" to these foods. Opiates, like opium, are highly addictive. If this "opiate excess" explanation applies to your child, then he is actually addicted to those foods containing the offending proteins. Although it seems as if your child will starve if you take those foods away, many parents report that after an initial "withdrawal" reaction, their children become much more willing to eat other foods. After a few weeks, most children surprise their parents by further broadening their diets.

Q: But if I take away milk, what will my child do for calcium?

A; Children between the ages of one and ten require 800-1000 mg of calcium/day. If the child drinks three 8oz glasses of fortified rice, soy or potato milk per day, he would meet that requirement. If he drank one cup per day the remaining 500 mg of additional calcium could be supplied with one of the many supplements available. Kirkman Labs (800-245-8282) makes flavored and flavorless calcium supplements in various forms. Custom-made calcium liquids can also be mixed up by compounding pharmacies using a maple, sucrose syrup, stevia or water base.

There are some very good calcium-enriched milk substitutes on the market. Rice Dream, in the white box, is usually available at the supermarket. Because this brand of rice milk is processed with barley enzymes, there is some concern over whether it will cause a reaction in individuals highly sensitive to gluten. layout child is also on a gluten-free diet, look for other brands of rice milk such as Pacific Foods, at your health food store. Darifree, a pleasant-tasting potato-based milk substitute which is lower in sugar than rice milk is available by mail-order (1-800-497-4834). Gluten-free soy milk is a good option for some, although many children with this disorder are intolerant to soy.

Q: Is this diet expensive?
A: There is no denying that some of the gluten-free ingredients you will want to keep on hand are more costly than the staples you are used to buying. However, when you order by the case, the above milk substitutes cost about the same as cow's milk. Some parents report that their autistic children were drinking over a gallon of cow's milk per day (about $60/month!) but these same parents were reluctant to switch to rice milk at $1.30/quart.

As with all foods convenience products such as frozen rice waffles are expensive, but making these from scratch is easy and inexpensive. Bulk rice flour is about 45c/pound, and there are several good gluten-free cookbooks. You'll find yourself making rice and potatoes more often, instead of ordering out. You might even save money.

Q: Isn't milk necessary for children's health?
A; Americans have been raised to believe that this is true, largely due to the efforts of the American Dairy Council, and many parents seem to believe that it is their duty to feed their children as much milk as possible.

However, lots of pefectly healthy children do very well without it. It's not milk that children need, it's calcium. Cow's milk has been called "the world's most overrated nutrient" and "fit only for baby cows." There is even evidence that the cow hormone present in dairy actually blocks the absorption of calcium in humans.

Be careful. Removing dairy means ALL milk, butter, cheese, cream cheese, sour cream, etc. It also includes product ingredients such as "casein" and "whey," or even words containing the word "casein." Read labels—items like bread and tuna fish often contain milk products. Even soy cheese usually contains caseinate.

For more information on dairy-free living, there's a very good book called *Raising Your Child Without Milk* by Jane Zukin. There is also a very good little book called *Don't Drink Your Milk* by Frank Oski (the late head of pediatrics at Johns Hopkins and author of *Essential Pediatrics*.)

This book cites the results of several research studies that conclude that milk is an inappropriate food for human children. It is available for $4.95 from Park City Press, PO Box 25, Glenwood Landing, NY 11547, ISBN #0671228048.

Q: I might be willing to try removing dairy products from his diet, but I don't think I could handle removing gluten. It seems like a lot of work, and I'm so busy already. Is this really necessary?
A: What you need to understand is that for certain children, these foods are toxic to their brains.

For some, removing gluten may be far more important than removing dairy products. You would never knowingly feed your child poison, but if he fits into this category, this is exactly what you could be doing. It is probable that for this subgroup of people with autism, eating these foods is actually damaging the developing brain.

Q: Removing both foods at once seems overwhelming. I'm afraid of my child's reaction. Can I start slowly?

A: Many parents strongly suggest that you try removing dairy first, and then work on planning for a completely gluten-free diet. Gluten can take more effort and some education on your part, and preparation may take a bit longer. Some physicians recommend doing this diet one step at a time to accurately record the child's response, and to reduce withdrawal reactions. The experts seem to agree that the milk and wheat proteins are so similar to each other that if one is a problem, the other should be removed as soon as possible.

Q: How do I know if this applies to my child?

A: Although there is some peptide testing available, there are many reports of false negatives and false positives. Widespread use of a reliable test is not yet available. DAN! Doctors and researchers agree that this is a very common problem in the autistic populaton, so a trial period on the diet may be your child's best bet. Although a lab result is more convincing to a doctor, the noticeable improvement many children exhibit will usually persuade even a reluctant spouse to support the diet.

Many affected children who eat a great deal of dairy and/or wheat-based foods will show changes within a few days of their elimination. For some, it can take up to three months. Some children don't appear to benefit significantly, yet when the proteins are reintroduced a regression is noted. The diet must be strict. Many parents have found that their child did not improve until they discovered and removed a hidden source of gluten or dairy. Noticeable changes in eye contact, sociability, and language are one sign that diet is an important issue. Another thing to look for are changes in the child's bowel movements or sleep patterns.

Q: When my child was taken just off dairy he improved greatly, but then he started eating a lot of wheat, perhaps to make up the opiates he was missing. Will I see the same kind of noticeable improvement when I remove gluten?
A: Children who eat a lot of gluten should show an improvement when it is removed. Some parents say that their child's response was more obvious with dairy, awesome with gluten. Gluten may take longer to disappear from the system than casein does. Urine tests show that casein probably leaves the system in about three days, but it might take up to eight months on a gluten-free diet for all peptide levels to drop. If this intervention is followed by a deterioration or regression (a withdrawal-type response), stay the course! It almost certainly means that your child will benefit. This may seem like a lot of work for an uncertain pay off, but in the lifetime of your child it may be the most important step you take.

Q: The only non-dairy, non-wheat foods my child will eat are french fries and chicken nuggets. Are these ok?
A: Chicken nuggets are coated with wheat. Some french fries are dusted with wheat flour to keep them from sticking together. It is a very good idea to get used to checking with your supplier or the manufacturer. Keeping a stack of blank pre-stamped postcards in the kitchen is a handy way to check.

The biggest problem with french fries eaten out of the house is contamination of the frying oil with gluten from onion rings and other breaded products. Making homemade fries is a good option. If your child refuses them at first, it may be because of what they're missing! Some parents report that their kids have an uncanny ability to detect gluten in foods. Since many of the children enjoy salt, salting the fries might make them more acceptable.

Q: What else contains gluten?
A: Wheat, oats, rye, barley, kamut, spelt, semolina, malt, food starch, grain alcohol, and most packaged foods—even those that do not label as such. There is a lot of information on gluten intolerance because of a related disorder called Celiac Disease.

Q: After I removed gluten and casein, I discovered that other foods seemed to be causing a problem, like apples, soy, corn, tomatoes, and bananas. I see irritability, red cheeks and ears, and sometimes diarrhea or a diaper rash. I thought you said that these kids don't have allergies!
A: Many do have allergies, or allergy-related symptoms such as hay fever, asthma or eczema.

Sometimes they have problems with foods which are not "classical" allergies, and which won't show up on skin tests. In this case, a different part of the immune system seems to be involved.

Q: So if these foods are not contributing to his autism, they're okay?
A: Not really. Current research indicates that in a great many cases, autism seems to be an immune system dysfunction. This can lead to a problem breaking down casein & gluten, but may also result in a problem breaking down phenolic foods (phenol sulfur transferals deficiency) and an over-reactive response to other allergens.

Often, once gluten is removed, this effect becomes more noticeable, perhaps because the allergens were "masked" by the effect of the gluten. It is also possible that a "Leaky gut syndrome," caused by the gluten intolerance, is now permitting other foods to pass through the intestinal screen and into the bloodstream.

For children who respond to this diet, allergens do seem to place further stress on the immune system, and have often been shown to worsen behavior and development.

Q: But my child's immune system seems to be working unusually well—he is rarely sick.
A; What we're describing is not an immune deficiency, but rather an immune dysfunction. Many (although not all) seem to share a history of fear infections and spitting up as babies (possibly milk-related) or of chronic diarrhea, constipation, or loose stools (possibly wheat-related). Other parents note that their autistic children seem to be the healthiest members of the family. In this case, it has been hypothesized that the immune system is too aggressive and ends up turning on the nervous system. This may explain the presence of anti-myelin antibodies in some children, and may also explain why some have immune issues like multiple allergies but do not respond well to dietary intervention.

Q: What causes this problem? Autism seems to be so much more common than it used to be.
A: Researchers are not sure, but it seems likely at this time that many cases are caused by a genetic predisposition or by environmental toxicity combined with some kind of triggering event that stresses the immune system, such as a vaccination

or virus. In several cases, prolonged use of antibiotics seems to have contributed to the onset of the disorder.

Q: So, if I can't give him milk or wheat, and if he has some other food allergies, what do I feed my child?
A: Most kids are okay with chicken, lamb, pork, fish, potato, rice, and egg whites. Parsnips, tapioca, arrowroot, honey, and maple syrup are usually okay too. French fries from McDonalds are currently gluten-free (but may contain soy or corn.) Certain white nuts, like macadamia and hazelnuts, are also usually tolerated. Others kids may be okay with white corn, bacon, frults such as white grapes or pears, beans, sesame seeds, or grains such as amaranth and teff (available at natural foods stores). There's always something to feed them—even the most finicky kids seem to like sticky white Chinese rice or fries.

Q: How do I know to which foods he's allerglc?
A: Try an allergy elimination diet. For example, keep common allergens out of his diet for a few days and then re-introduce them, one-by-one. If you see symptoms, either physical or behavioral, try again in a few days. Try to be systematic, to be certain before ruling out a food. Two excellent resources, probably available at your library are Doris Rapp's book, *Is This Your Child*, and William Crook's *Solving the Puzzle of Your Hard to Raise Child*.

Q: I'm already worried about my child's nutrition, and his "allergies" are causing me to further reduce his choices. If apple juice and bananas are the only fruits he will eat and he's reacting to them, how is he supposed to get by?
A: Fruit contains water, sugar, fiber, and vitamins. He needs to get these things from other sources.

Q: I thought the "five food groups" were so important!
A: They are, to an individual without food intolerances. But, just as a person who eats a balanced diet might not need to take vitamins, one with poor nutrition can make up for a lot with a good vitamin and mineral supplement.

Q: So I should be giving my child a vitamin supplement?
A: Absolutely. Poly-vi-sol with Iron is probably okay to start with, or order a gluten-free multivitamin & mineral formula from your natural foods store. Kal Dinosaur Chewables and "I Love Schiff" liquid and chewables are tolerated by many food-sensitive children, and are available with or without minerals.

Because many autistic children have been reported to improve on a regimen of vitamin B6 and magnesium, you may want to order supplement rich in these nutrients from a lab such as Kirkman (800-245-8282). For a 40 pound child, Dr Bernard Rimland of the Autism Research Institute recommends 300 mgs. of B6 and 100 mgs. of magnesium per day. It is likely that in people with a leaky gut, absorption of B6 (which aids in nervous system function) is often greatly diminished.

Q: What else does my child need?
A: There are six basic things a person needs from food: water, protein (and amino acids), carbohydrates, fats, vitamins, minerals (including iron & calcium). In addition, food contains certain photochemical substances that seem to help with functions like disease prevention. It is helpful to consult a nutritionist about the use of supplements such as pycnogenol for any child on a limited diet.

Children who have gone for one year eating only chicken, canola oil, potato, rice, calcium-enriched beverages and a liquid multivitamin supplement with minerals have had excellent results on nutritional blood tests. You'd be surprised to learn just how unnecessarily varied an American diet is, compared with the diets of other cultures!

Q: So how do I know if my child will respond to this diet?
A: The biggest clue is when a child self-limits his diet—especially to milk and wheat. This is no longer seen as a "need for sameness" but as a biological addiction. Children who don't necessarily "self-limit" but who also respond are those who eat an unusually large or small amount of food. Although the former may not recognize the source of the opiates, he knows that eating makes him feel GOOD. The latter may realize that many foods make him feel ill, and tries to avoid eating whenever possible. These "failure to thrive" autistic children are very hard to put on this diet because of their parents' fears, but will usually respond when acceptable substitutes to the non-tolerated foods can be provided.

Other symptoms of food intolerance or vitamin deficiency are dermatitis or extremely dry skin, migraines, bouts of screaming, red cheeks, red ears, abnormal bowel movements, abnormal sleep patterns or seizures.

Q: What's all this I hear about yeast?
A: Candida and other yeasts live in our bodies in small amounts. It was speculated that in individuals with improperly-functioning immune systems, they could flourish in the gut and lead to a host of problems, including fatigue, sugar cravings, headaches, and behavioral problems.

Q: How do we know if this is really true?

A: We didn't until recently. Dr William Shaw in Kansas found unusually high levels of "fungal metabolites" (yeast waste products) in the urine of several groups of abnormally functioning individuals (including people with autism). His first paper describing this phenomenon was published in the *Journal of Clinical Chemistry* in 1995 (Vol. 41, No. 8). His urinary organic acids test is performed by the Great Plains exploratory (913-341-8949).

Q: So does yeast cause autism?

A: This finding may be just another consequence of the abnormally-functioning autistic immune system. However, early antibiotic use may actually be the triggering factor for children predisposed to autism. It has been hypothesized that the candida might aggravate a condition of gut permeability (the "leaky gut" syndrome) which might let the gluten and casein proteins into the bloodstream before they are broken down, so it may in part be responsible for autistic behaviors. Many parents of children with ADD/ADHD as well as those with autism report that treatment for candida does improve their children's behavior and concentration.

Q: How do I treat for candida?

A: One approach is to ask your pediatrician for a course of Nystatin, which is a non-systemic (not absorbed into the bloodstream) anti-fungal. Taken orally it works locally in the gut to fight candida.

This medication is considered to be quite safe, even when taken for several months. For a 25-35 lb. child, ask the doctor for a prescription for Nystatin powder (125,000 units per cc) in a stevia base, starting with 1 cc 4x/day. Your local pharmacy probably carries a commercial preparation in a sugar base—this feeds yeast! Try a compounding pharmacy such as Pathway (800-869-9160).

"Probiotics" such as acidophilus, the natural bacteria found in yogurt, are other candida fighters and are available at the natural foods store in powdered form in the refrigerated section. Some acidophilus preparations are milk-based—be sure to get one that is not! Bifidus works in the large intestine and can be of great benefit. "FOS" is desirable in these supplements, as it feeds the probiotics.

Q: Aren't probiotics the "healthy flora" I've heard about?
A: Yes, they compete with candida for the sugars you eat. It's the "good bacteria." You may be aware that acidophilus is eradicated from your gut when you take antibiotics.

Q: My friend's child tried Nystatin and it made him vomit. If Nystatin is so safe, why did he react to it?
A: The child may have experienced a "die-off reaction" to the candida. As it dies, candida releases toxins into the bloodstream and can cause nausea, vomiting, or diarrhea. It is likely that candida was indeed a problem for this child. Your friend should discuss a dosage change (starting with a low dose and working up to a "normal dose") with the prescribing doctor.

Q: My doctor has never heard of any of this and she is extremely skeptical. I'm embarrassed to tell her I'm considering this approach.
A: Skepticism is a good thing in a medical doctor or scientist. However, since there is preliminary evidence to support this safe, non-invasive intervention, it is up to you to educate her,

state your wishes, and ask for her support. For a doctor, it is better to wait until all of the data is published in peer-reviewed journals before advocating a treatment. For a parent, it is reasonable to want to help one's child without waiting for all of the results of the "double-blind placebo" studies. Because this approach does not include any unusual supplements, invasive drugs, or expensive treatments, your pediatrician should be supportive. Explain that you would like to try this for a few weeks, and agree that you will be objective about recording your child's progress while on the diet.

Q: Where can I find support?

A: It is likely that other parents in your area are already aware of this intervention. Ask your local chapter of the ASA for the nearest dietary intervention support group, or form one yourself. There are also several support groups for the biological treatment of autism on the Internet (search "Autism and Diet," as well as support for a gluten-free diet (search "Celiac Disease"). A valuable resource is The ANDI News. To subscribe to the ANDI Newsletter, send $20 ($26 for subscriptions outside of the U.S.). Include your name & address, clearly printed. Mail orders to:

The Autism Network for Dietary Intervention

PO Box 17711 Rochester, NY 14617-0711

Appendix IV
DoingYour Own Research by "Surfing the Net"

With a computer, a (relatively high speed) modem and some software, you have a wealth of information at your fingertips. With these three things, you will have access to the Internet, the so-called "Information Superhighway," as well as to electronic mail and news groups on every subject imaginable. Electronic mail alone would make these purchases worthwhile; it provides nearly instantaneous contact with people around the world who share your interests.

If you have a computer but no modem, visit your local computer store and find out what type will be compatible with your computer. Buy the fastest modem you can afford (they are relatively inexpensive). Modem speed is measured in "baud" rate—try to buy one that is at least 56,600.

The baud rate measures how many computer "bits per second" are transferred over your phone connection. A slow connection will make it too cumbersome to read large files.

Once you have the right hardware, you must choose the software you will use to communicate with the world. Some of the more popular vendors are America Online (AOL), Compuserve and Prodigy. Most of these companies offer free trials. I would suggest you get several of the trial accounts and determine which you like best. If you have recently purchased a computer that came with Windows98® as its operating system, then you need not buy extra software. Windows98® comes complete with software for reaching the Internet.

Perhaps the most popular aspect of the Internet, is what is known as the "World Wide Web" (AKA the WWW or The Web). People all over the world have published documents, known as "pages" or "home pages" on the Web. Using special software (available with your Internet Provider software) called "search engines," you can reach these pages in a matter of seconds. When you find a page that interests you, it will likely lead you to other, related pages via "hot links." You know a word or set of words is a link if it is underlined (generally in a different color than the rest of the text); clicking your mouse button on such a link instantly transports you to it, even if it is residing on a computer thousands of miles away.

Before you know it, you will be exploring thousands of computers with millions of pages of information. The "search engine" software will allow you to look for subjects that interest you; each page reference that is returned in response to your search is called a "hit."

As stated above web pages are reached by "clicking" a word or phrase; these "clickable" words are linked to an odd looking sentence that typically begins with "www...". These sentences are actually addresses, known as URLs (Universal Resource Locators). If you read magazines or watch television, you have no doubt seen such URLs. Nearly every advertisement has, in small print, the URL for that company's web page (e.g. during a commercial for a Toyota Camry you'll see www.toyota.com displayed at the bottom of your television screen). Often, you can make an educated guess about what a URL will be. They almost always start with "www". Companies will then have their name, generally followed by ".com" (which stands for commercial). Government pages will end in ".gov". Educational institutions end in ".edu" and, nonprofit organization addresses typically end in ".org".

This information will allow you to begin exploring the net. Using the search engines provided by your Internet software is another, perhaps more systematic way of finding information. To get you started, I will list some URLs likely to be of interest. Nearly every one of them provides many hot links to other, related pages, and should keep you happily surfing for many, many hours! In addition to surfing around the Web, the Internet has many news groups. Most Internet software will also allow you to access news groups. It will allow you to subscribe to a particular group, and then read all the postings to it. When a subscriber "posts" to the list, he is writing a single message that is available to every subscriber to the group. Once posted, other subscribers can reply to it publicly (i.e. to the whole list) or send a reply to the writer of the article. There are many lists about topics of yeast, autism, add/adhd and other disabilities. Your software will allow you to look at the names of all available groups and choose those you wish to view regularly. You can also set most software to alert you when new groups are available.

The amount of information that is available to you, once you have the proper hardware and software, is staggering. It increases daily and so far, there is no end in sight. Perhaps as important as what you will learn, is how many people there are out there in the same boat. There is much to learn, and much to share.

One important warning about the WWW: There is no control over who publishes what.

Resources may be well-written and sound authoritative, but if the source is an organization or individual you have never heard of, be sure to find other supporting sources before taking the contents as accurate. Anyone can say they have credentials but there is little that you can do to check them. This does not detract from the fact that there is a huge amount of excellent and useful information out there—it simply means that you need to always "consider the source." This is good advice in general and certainly important when you are doing Internet research. Good luck and happy surfing!

Web Pages of Interest

Pages on ADHD

PAR is short for Parents Against Ritalin. An active group, they run several related sites and can be found at their home page:

www.p-a-r.org/

Children and Adults with Attention Deficit Disorder is a national organization which is supposed to be a good source of information about living with and treating ADD. Beware however-CHADD asserts that Ritalin is the only useful treatment for this disorder. Not exactly a surprise since the group is largely funded by Ciba-Geigy, the makers of Ritalin!

www.chadd.org

Dr. Allen Buresz has a web page entitled: "Success With Attention Deficit Disorder and Hyperactivity." This page discusses non-drug alternatives, and has many interesting links.

www.all-natural.com/add.html

Pages on Autism Spectrum Disorders and Related Topics

John Wobus, the parent of an autistic child, maintains an excellent site at Syracuse University. This site contains the most complete list of autism and related links that I have ever come across. This is the place to start:

www.vaporia.com/autism

An excellent page about Asperger syndrome by people who should know contributors have AS or are HFAs.

http://amug.org/~a203/

The Center for Autism home page includes links to many valuable sources on information and articles, including links to Bernard Rimland's Autism Research International and Jaak Panksepp's Memorial Foundation for Lost Children.

www.autism.com

Autism Books and Publications run by Future Horizons, this site allows online ordering of books, audiotapes of conferences and videotapes of interest. Be sure to check this site out from time to time, as offerings change. Also includes listings of upcoming conferences.

http://www.futurehorizons-autism.com

O.A.S.I.S stands for Online Asperger Syndrome Information and Support. Their home page has many good links and articles.

www.udel.edu/bkirby/asperger/

The Autism Research Unit is the web page of Paul Shattock's group at the University of Sunderland.

http://osiris.sunderland.ac.uk/autism/

Allergy Induced Autism is a group formed several years ago in England. It was this group that encouraged Rosemary Waring's research on PST deficiency and its possible association with autism.

www.demon.co.ukcharities/AIA/aia.htm

The Great Plains Laboratory will send you a collection kit for testing your child's urine for organic acids (i.e. fungal metabolites). Call them at 913-341-8949 or visit their website to order kits.

www.greatplainslaboratory.com

Dr. Sidney Baker maintains a very useful website with resources and information pertinent to autism:

www.sbakermd.com

Dr. Jeff Bradstreet maintains a website with very good information about autism treatment.

http://www.gnd.org

Therapeutic Play for Children and Their Parents is a site which contains many ideas for using play therapy.

http://www.theraplay.org

The Developmental Delay Resources (DDR) is a nonprofit organization concerned with developmental delays in sensory motor, language, social and emotional areas. They publish research and provide a network for parents and professionals. Their newsletter tracks current research and trends.

www.devdelay.org

The HANDLE Institute "provides drug-free alternatives for identifying and treating most neurodevelopmental disorders across the life span." They use research and techniques from medicine, rehabilitation, psychology, education and nutrition.

www.handle.org

Pages on Special Diets

Don Wiss is a celiac who maintains an excellent site on many diet related topics. Interested in the connection between gluten and autism, parents of autistic children with food allergies or intolerances will find his pages extremely useful.

www.panix.com/donwiss *see also* **www.panix.com/nomilk**

When an Internet list was created on the topic of Celiac, it soon had many subscribers, including many parents of autistic children. The list later made its posts available via news groups, which can be accessed by anyone with a modem, an Internet Service Provider, and newsreader software.

Archives of the Celiac news group have been indexed and stored on a web site, and these articles are excellent sources anyone living with dietary restrictions.

http://www.fastlane.net/homepages/thodge/archive.htm

The most complete list of gfcf foods can be found at: **www.gfcfdiet.com.** It is a MUST VISIT location.

What's In a Label? This is the question answered by this web site, which demystifies the labels now required on every food sold in this country.

www.fda.gov/fdac/special/foodlabel/ingred.html

Product Alerts are released to various consumer groups, whenever ingredients have been recalled, or when a change in ingredients renders it unsafe for a particular group. This site will help keep individuals abreast of such changes.

www.foodallergy.org/alerts.html

The Feingold Association maintains a very good page, well worth a visit to:

www.feingold.org

My own page contains my original article on the subject covered in this book, pictures of my children, and a list of links that I think are useful to those with interests in dietary intervention.

http://members.aol.com/lisas156/index.htm

Along with K. Seroussi, I have begun publication of a quarterly newsletter ("The ANDI News") on the subject of dietary intervention for autism. The newsletter contains research updates, recipes, conference announcements and cooking tips. For questions and subscription requests write to: AutismNDI@aol.com

www.AutismNDI.com

Many people write to me asking about support groups. There is an online list you may find useful. Go to **www.onelist.com** and search on GFCFkids. This is an online "community" that you will find very helpful.

Pages on Special Education

For information about writing IEPs, go to:

http://www.autism-society.org/packages/IEP.html

Pages on "Alternative" Treatments and Medicine

Mothers for Natural Law—a page about the dangers of vaccines and other medical practices.

http://www.safe-food.org/welcome.html

If you are interested in learning more about the overgrowth of yeast, look at these pages:

http://members.aol.com/docdarren/med/candida.html

**http://www.mall-net.com/arth1.html
(about arthritis and candida)**

http://www.healthexcel.com/docs/ candl.html (yeast)

http://www.panix.com|-candida/

www.yeastconnection.com (Dr. William Crook's site)

Pages on Funding Organizations

An excellent and complete page by "Cure Autism Now," an organization devoted to raising funds for autism research.

http://www.canfoundation.org

Home page of the National Organization for Autism Research-NAAR

http://www.naar.org

Pages On Finding Medical Information, Supplements, Drugs

The Apothecary is a Maryland "compounding pharmacy," that is, they can prepare supplements and medicines according to the doctor's instructions (or that of a parent if it is for a non-prescription item such as vitamins and minerals). This pharmacy will use flavorings that are acceptable for your child.

www.the-apothecary.com/

MSB: Psychopharmacologic and Neurologic (CNS) Drug Reviews. Though we all aim to avoid drugs for our children, there are times when symptoms cannot be dealt with in other ways. This site provides good information on various medications that may be suggested.

www.pharminfo.com/

PubMed is a wonderful Internet resource. In the past, access to the best medical reference and abstracting service (Medscape) was expensive to use and required a subscription. Now, thanks to an initiative by former Vice President Al Gore, anyone in the world can have free access to this particular website.

www.ncbi.nlm.nih.gov/pubmed

Stokes Pharmacy, in Medford, NJ, is an excellent source of information about the gluten and dairy status of prescription and otc medications.

www.stokesRx.com

For information about vaccine safety, contact the National Vaccine Information Center (NVIC) at 800-909-SHOT or visit

www.909shot.com

The Autism Autoimmunity Project is online at

www.gti.net/truegrit

Appendix V
Other Cookbooks

Parents often call or write to me with the question: "Where should I start?" I often answer "at the library." I have used libraries all my life, but it was only recently that I realized that libraries usually have extensive cookbook selections.

Until you have cooked from a book, it is hard to know whether the recipes in it will be ones your family enjoys. Using the library allows you to experiment with recipes, read recipes to get an idea of whether or not they sound good, contain allowed ingredients or will permit substitutions—all without having to buy the book. Look for a section on Special Diets. Pick carefully. Many times a book removing particular ingredients (e.g. a dairy-free cookbook) will contain recipes that are also gluten-free.

Look through the ethnic cookbook section very carefully. There are many good choices there. Look at cuisines you might not have ever thought of cooking; Korean food is delicious, and almost completely rice based. Other nationalities will also offer you new choices.

After you have checked out a number of cookbooks, you should have a good idea of what books to buy. Obviously, if a book only has three recipes you think your family would like, it makes sense to copy those and skip that one on your trip to the bookstore. But there will certainly be cookbooks you will want to own. If your local store does not have a good selection of specialty or ethnic cookbooks, you might want to visit Amazon

Books on the Internet. This is a cyber-bookstore that offers millions of titles. Once you have registered, you can browse and shop from your own home. Amazon even keeps track of what books you have ordered in the past, and lets you know when a new book is published that may be of interest to you! To find them, go to **http://www.amazon.com**.

The list that follows is certainly not exhaustive—it is merely a selection of some of my favorite cookbooks. Many (most) are not exclusively GF, but all have wonderful recipes that can at least be the starting point for a delicious meal.

Cookbooks

The Candida Control Cookbook, by Gail Burton (1993). Published by Aslan Publishing.

The Complete Allergy Self-Help Cookbook, by Marjorie Hurt Jones, R.N. (1984). Published by Rodale Press.

The Complete Food Allergy Cookbook, *The Foods You've Always Loved Without the Ingredients You Can't Have*, by Marilyn Gioannini (1995). Published by Prima Pub.

Delicious & Easy Rice Flour Recipes: Coping with the GF Diet by Marion N. Wood (1972). Published by Charles C Thomas Pub Ltd.

Dietary Intervention as a Therapy in the Treatment of Autism and Related Developmental Disorders by Beth and Andy ⸻ (1995).

⸻ *Bread Making for Special Diets* by Nicolette Dumke ⸻. Adapt Books: Louisville, CO.

"The Gluten-Free Baker Newsletter" by Sandra Leonard, 361 Cherrywood Dr., Fairborn, OH 45324-4012, e-mail: thebaker@CRIS.COM.

Gluten-Free Dessert Cookbook, c/o Designer Interiors, 3270 CamdenRue, Cuyahoga Falls, OH 44223, $19.95, e-mail: designerinteriors@MSN.com

http://www.inc.com/users/COOKBOOK.html

The Gluten-Free Gourmet by Betty Hagman, (1991). Published by Henry Holt (Paper).

The Gluten-Free Gourmet Cooks Fast and Healthy: Wheat-Free and Gluten-Free With No Fuss and Less Fat, by Bette Hagman, (1996). Published by Henry Holt (Paper).

Going Against the Grain, by Phyllis Potts, (1992). Published by Central Point Publishing.

Jane Brody's Good Food Book: Living the High Carbohydrate Way, by Jane E. Brody, (1985). Published by W. W. Norton & Co.

More from the Gluten-Free Gourmet: Delicious Dining Without Wheat by Bette Hagman, (1994). Published by Henry Holt (Paper).

The No-Gluten Solution: Children Cookbook, (1991). by Pat Cassady Redjou. Published by Rae Pub.

Still Going Against the Grain, by Phyllis Potts (1994). Published by Central Point Publishing.

Still Life With Menu Cookbook by Mollie Katzen, (1994). Published by Ten Speed Press.

The Wheat-Free Kitchen. A Celebration of Good Foods by Jacqueline Mallorca, Farthing Press, PO Box 471171, San Francisco, CA 94147.

Other Helpful Resources

The CSA/USA sells a shopping guide. The cost is $8.00 and lists 39 categories of products. To order, send check payable to: CSA/USA, Inc. PO Box 31700, Omaha, NE 58131-0700.

Another gluten and casein-free shopping guide can be ordered for $10.00. Send request with check to: TCCSSG Shopping Guide, 34638 Beechwood, Farmington Hills, MI 48335. Put this to the attention of Ms. Marcia Campbell.

References

(1) Baker, S. M. (1997) *Detoxification and Healing: The Key to Optimal Health.* Keats Publishing Company, Inc.: New Cannas, CT.

(2) Barkley, R.,A. and J.V. Murphy (1991) *"Treating Attention Deficit Hyperactivity Disorder: Medication and Behavior Management Trainings," Pediatric Annals*, 20:26-66.

(3) Bernard, Betty (1993) "Gluten Sensitive Disorders: Celiac Disease (CD) and Dermatitis Herpetiformis (DH). Synopsis: Celiac Disease." *Publication of the American Celiac Society.*

(4) Bock S. A. and F. M. Atkins (1990) Conclusions of 1990 article reprinted by the International Food Information Council in *Food Insight*, May/lune 1991 issue.

(5) Boris, M. and F.S. Mandel (1994) "Foods and additives are common causes of attention deficit hyperactive disorder in children." *Ann. Allergy*, 72 (5) 462-468.

(6) Bjarneson, I., A. MacPherson and D. Hollander (1995) "Intestinal Permeability: An Overview" *Gastroenterology*, 108:1566-1581.

(7) Braverman, E., Carl C. Pfeiffer, Ken Blumb, Richard Smayda (1997) *The Healing Nutrients Within: Facts, Findings and New Research on Amino Acids*, 2nd edition. Keats Publishing: New Cannas, CT.

(8) Campbell, M. E. Schopler, J.E. Cueva, Al Hallin (1996) "Treatment of Autistic Disorder." *J. Amer. Acad. Child and Adolesc. Psych.*, 35:134-143.

(9) Catassi, C., I-M Ratsch, E. Fabiani, M. Rossini, F. Bordicchia, F. Candela, G.V. Coppa and P.L. Giorgi (1994). "Coeliac disease in the year 2000: exploring the iceberg," *The Lancet*, Vol. 343: 188-203.

(10) Coll, D.A., C.A. Rosen, K. Auborn, W. Potsic and H.L. Bradlow (1997). "Treatment of Recurrent Respiratory Papillomatosis with Indole-3-Carbinol," *Amer.J. of Otolaryng.* Vol. 18, No. 4, pp 283-285.

(11) Comings, David E., M.D. (1990) *Tourette's Syndrome and Human Behavior*. Duarte, California, Hope Press.

(12) Crook, W. (1986) *The Yeast Connection*, Professional Books: Jackson, TN.

(13) ____(1990) *Tracking Down Hidden Food Allergies*. Professional Books: Jackson, TN.

(14) D'Eufemia, P., M. Celli, R. Finocchiaro, L. Pacifico, L. Viozzi, L. Zaccagnin, E. Cardi, P. Giardini (1996) "Abnormal Intestinal Permeability in Children with Autism." *Acta Paediatrica*, 85:1076-79.

(15) Dohan, F.C. (1966) "Cereals and Schizophrenia—Data and Hypothesis." *Acta Psychiatr. Scand* 42:125

(16) _____(1976) "The Possible Pathogenic Effect of Cereal Grains in Schizophrenia Celiac Disease as a Model." *Acta Neurol*. 31:195.

(17) Dorfman, K. (1997) "Improving Detoxification Pathways," in *New Developments*, Vol. 2, No. 3. pp. 4.

(18) Edelson, Stephen B. (1997) A series of informational articles available from the Environmental and Preventive Health Center of Atlanta website: http://www.ephca.com

(19) Feingold, Ben (1975) *Why Your Child is Hyperactive*. Random House: New York.

(20) Freeman. John M., M.D., Millicent T. Kelly, Jennifer B. Freeman (1996) *The Epilepsy Treatment: An Introduction to the Ketogenic Diet*, 2nd edition. Demos Publications: New York.

(21) Freeman, John M. (1997) "Statement of the Child Neurology Society on The Ketogenic Diet" Published on the Internet by the Child Neurology Society, http://www.umn.edu/cns/ ketodiet.html.

(22) Fukudome, S-I and M. Yoshikawa (1992). "Opiod peptides derived from wheat gluten: their isolation and characterization," *Federation of European Biochemical Societies,* Vol. 296, No. 1.: 107-111.

(23) Galland, Leo M.D., Dian Dincin Buchman (1989) *Superimmunity For Kids.* Reissued by Delacourte Press.

(24) Gardner, Robert W. (1994). *Chemical Intolerance.* CRC Press, Inc.: Boca Raton.

(25) Gillberg, C. (1988) "The role of endogenous opioids in autism and possible relationships to clinical features" in Wing, L. (ed.) *Aspects of Autism: Biological Research.* Gaskell: London, pp. 31-37.

(26) Gottschall, Elaine. (1994) *Breaking the Vicious Cycle: Intestinal Health Through Diet.* Kirkton, Ont.: Kirkton Press.

(27) Green, Michael (1994) "RRP Research News: Treatment Protocols and Cabbage Juice Recipes." *Recurrent Respiratory Papillomatosis Newsletter*, Vol. 3 No. 2. RRP Foundation Publication: Lawrenceville, NJ.

(28) Horrobin, David.(1981) *Journal of Holistic Medicine*, Vol. 3, No. 2, Winter, pp.132.

(29) Johnson, S. (1995) "Sara's Diet," a private publication available from PO Box 939, Glen Alpine, North Carolina 28628. (Write for information and fees.)

(30) Kakuta, Kazuhiko, M.D. (1992) "Utilizing Whale Meat To Overcome Food Allergies." *Isama*, Vol. 7.

(31) Knivsberg, A-M., Wiig, K., Lind, G., Nodland, M., Reichelt, L.L (1990) "Dietary Interventions in Autistic Syndromes," *Brain Dysfunction*, 3: (5-6): 315-327.

(32) _____, K. Reichelt, M. Nodland, G. Lind (1994) "Probable Etiology and Possible Treatment of Childhood Autism." *Brain Dysfunction*, 4:308-19.

(33) Kummel, D. (1996) "Lipids," in: *Krause's Food, Nutrition and Diet Therapy*. L.K. Mahan *et. al.* (eds.)

(34) Lapchick, J. Michael and Cindy Appleseth, R.Ph. (1993) *The Label Reader's Pocket Dictionary of Food Additives*. Chronomed Publishing: Minneapolis, MN.

(35) McFadden, S. A. (1996) "Phenotypic variation in xenobiotic metabolism and adverse environmental response: focus on self-dependent detoxification pathways." *Toxicology*, 111(1-3): 43-65.

(36) Mindell, E. (1992) *Earl Mindell's Herb Bible*. Simon and Schuster, New York.

(37)___(1992) *Parent's Nutrition Bible: A Guide to Raising Healthy Children*. Hay House: Carson, CA.

(38) Nsouli, T.M., Lind, S.M., Linde, R.E., O'Mara, F., Scanlon, R.T. and Bellanti, J.A. (1994). "Role of food allergy in serious otitis media," *Annals of Allergy*, 73(3): 215-9.

(39) O'Reilly, B. A. and R.H. Waring (1993) "Enzyme and Sulphur Oxidation Deficiencies in Autistic Children with Known Food/Chemical Intolerances." *J. Orthomolec. Med*, 8 (4) 198-200.

(40) Oski, Frank A. (1992) Don't Drink Your Milk!: New Frightening Medical Facts About the World's Most Overrated Nutrient, Rh Edition. Teach Services: Boston, NY.

(41) Panksepp, J. (1979.) "A neurochemical theory of autism." *Trends in Neuroscience*, 2: 174-177.

(42) Panksepp, J., Herman, B. H. , Villberg, T. , Bishop, P. and DeEskinazi, F. G. (1980). "Endogenous opioids and social behavior." *Neuroscience and Biobehavioral Reviews*, 4, 473-487.

(43) Pfeiffer, S.L., J. Norton, L. Nelson and S. Shott (1995) "Efficacy of Vitamin B6 and Magnesium in the Treatment of Autism: A Methodology Review and summary." *J Aut. Dev. Dis.* 25:481-493.

(44) Rapp, Doris, M.D. (1991) *Is This Your Child? Discovering and Treating Unrecognized Allergies in Children and Adults.* William Morrow: New York.

(45) Reichelt, K.L., J. Ekrem, H. Scot (1990) "Gluten, Milk Proteins and Autism: Dietary Intervention Effects on Behavior and Peptide Secretion." *Journal of Applied Nutrition* 42 (1):1-11.

(46) Reichelt, K.L., K. Hole, A. Hamburger, G. Saelid, P.D. Edminson, C.B. Braestrup, O. Lingjaerde, P. Ledaal, H. Orbeck (1981). "Biologically Active Peptide Containing Fractions in Schizophrenia and Childhood Autism." *Adv. Biochem. Psychopharmacol.* 28:27-643.

(47) Reichenberg-Ullman, J. and R. Ullman (1996) *Ritalin-Free Kids,* Prima Publishing: Rocklin, CA.

(48) Rimland, B. and D. I. Meyer (1967) "Malabsorption and the Celiac Syndrome as Possible Causes of Childhood Psychosis: A Brief Discussion of Evidence and Needed Research".

(49) Rona, Zoltan P. (1997) "Hidden Hazards of Vitamin and Mineral Tablets." Published on WWW at: *http://www.naturallink.com.*

(50) Rosenvold, L. M.D. (1992) *Can a Gluten-Free Diet Help? How?* New Caanan, CT, Keats Publishing.

(51) Rowe, K.S. and K.J. Rowe (1994) "Synthetic food coloring and behavior: a dose response effect in a double-blind, placebo-controlled, repeated-measures study." *J Pediatr.* 125 (5 Pt 1): 691-698.

(52) Schmidt, M.A., L.H. Smith, K.W. Sehnert (1993) *Beyond Antibiotics: 50 (or so) Ways to Boost Immunity and Avoid Antibiotics.* North Atlantic Books: Berkeley, CA.

(53) Shattock, P., A. Kennedy, F. Rowell and T. Bernet (1990). "Role of Neuropeptides in Autism and Their Relationships with Classical Neurotransmitters." *Brain Dysfunction*, Vol 3:328-345.

(54) , Lowdon, G. (1991) "Proteins, Peptides and Autism. Part 2: Implications for the Education and Care of People with Autism," *Brain Dysfunction*, 4 (6) 323-334.

(55)_____(1995) "Back To the Future: An assessment of some of the unorthodox forms of biomedical intervention currently being applied to autism," Psychological Perspectives in Autism: Collected papers from the conference organised by the autism Research Unit, University of Sunderland, pp. 195-202.

(56)_____, and D. Savery (1997) "Evaluation of Urinary Profiles Obtained from People with Autism and Associated Disorders. Part 1: Classification of Subgroups. Unpub. Ms.

(57) Shaw, W., Kassen, E. (1995) "Increased Urinary Excretion of Analogs of Krebs Cycle Metabolites and Arabinose in Two Brothers with Autistic Features." *Clin. Chem.*, Vol. 41 (8), pp. 1094-1104.

(58)____(1998) *Biological Treatments for Autism and PDD.*

(59) Siegel, B. (1996) *The World of the Autistic Child.* Oxford University Press: New York.

(60) Sinaiko, R.J. (1996) "The Biochemistry of Attentional/ Behavioral Problems." Paper presented at the 1996 Feingold Association Conference in Orlando, Florida.

(61) Stern, William (1997) "Adjunct Therapy and Protocol Update," *Recurrent Respiratory Papillomatosis Newsletter*, Vol. 6 No.1. RRP Foundation Publication: Lawrenceville, NJ.

(62) Sullivan, R. C. (1975) "Hunches on Some Biological Factors in Autism," *J. of Autism And Childhood Schiz*, Vol. 5, No. 2. pp. 177-184.

(63) Travathan, E. (1996) "The Ketogenic Diet—Does It Work In Children?" *Epilepsy Update*, No. 6.

(64) Wallis, C. (1994) "An Epidemic of Attention Deficit Disorder." *Time*, 144:42-50.

(65) Waring, R.H. and Ngong, J.M. (1993) "Sulphate Metabolism in Allergy-Induced Autism: Relevance to the Disease Aetiology," Conference papers from: Biological Perspectives in Autism, held at the University of Durham, April, 1993. Published by Autism Research Unit, University of Stmderland. 25-33.

(66) _____, Reichelt, K. (1996) "The Biochemistry of the Autistic Syndrome" in *Autism on the Agenda*. P. Shattock and G. Linfoot (eds.) NAS, London, pp. 125-127.

(67) Williams, K., P. Shattock, T. Berney (1991) "Proteins, Peptides and Autism: Part 1: Urinary Protein Patterns in Autism as Revealed by Sodium Dodecyl Sulphate-polyacrylamide Gel Electrophoresis and Silver Staining." *Brain Dysfunction*, 4:320-22.

Gluten-Free & Casein-Free Resources

Web Pages on Dietary Intervention

Autism Network for Dietary Intervention:
http://www.AutismNDI.com **-Information & links**

GFCF Kids: http://www.gfcfdiet.com
Contains good information AND a list of brand-name products! You can also join a discussion group for parents implementing this diet—a wonderful resource.

www.panix.com/~donwiss
A great site that links to many other gf/cf sites.

www.fastlane.net/homepages/thodge/archive.html
The archives of the WWW Celiac listserv.

Dr. Jeff Bradstreet: http://www.gnd.orc

Sidney M. Baker, M.D. http://www.sbakermd.com

For more general information about autism with lots of useful links: http://www.autism.org

Web-Based Mail Order Resources

American Spoon Foods sells sauces, salad dressings, jams, "spoon fruit" and tart dried cherries, sweetened only by concentrated juices.

http://www.spoon.com

Authentic Foods. Their bread, cookie, cake and other mixes are made with flour that is a combination of garbanzo (chickpea) and lava beans. You can also buy the flours and make your own.

htp://www.authenticfoods.com

The Chocolate Emporium sells Kosher chocolate and other candy. Many are dairy-free and some are also gluten-free. They can tell you which candies are acceptable. Be sure to put in a big order around the Jewish holiday of Passover (in March or April) when an even larger assortment is available.

http://www.choclat.com

Dietary Specialties: This company carries many baking ingredients, mixes, snacks, pastas etc. They even carry condiments, such as pickles, mustard and various sauces.

http://www.dietspec.com

Ener-G Foods sells xanthan gum and many other ingredients. Their "GF Gourmet Blend" is the Hagman GF flour mix—sold in one pound pouches or 5 pound bags. They also sell baked goods, but their breads are not as good as others listed here.

www.ener-g.com

Food for Life Baking Co. has a site that sells their breads and banana muffins online, and also has a search facility to find a retailer near you. People particularly like the pecan rice and almond rice loaf.

http://www.food-for-life.com

Gifts of Nature sells a GF flour blend that is a one-for-one substitute for flour in any recipe. They specialize in baking mixes made with brown rice and bean flours.

www.giftsofnature.hypermart.net

The Gluten-Free Mall claims to be a "one-stop shop" on the Internet for gluten-free and wheat-free products. The Mall combines the complete catalogues of different gluten-free food companies, but orders are actually placed individually with each company, so shipping cost are high if an order is from multiple vendors.

http://www.glutenfreemall.com

The Gluten-Free Pantry is known for its excellent mixes for breads, cookies and pancakes, cakes, bagels, baking ingredients and more. Some mixes are sold in health food stores, but the full line is available only through mail order. Some mixes contain dairy, so read labels carefully.

http://www.glutenfree.com/index.html

Jowar Foods sells sorghum based food products. Site includes information, products, and recipes.

http://www.jowar.com

King Arthur Flour sells primarily wheat-based products, but they also carry tapioca flour, white rice flour, potato starch flour and xanthan gum. They carry hard to find baking utensils (e.g. hot dog and hamburger bun pans). A good source for additive-free dehydrated egg whites and meringue powder.

http://www.kingarthurflour.com

Kinnikinnick Foods is a Canadian company has many good baked items, plus ingredients. Kinnikinnick is one of the few places that stocks rice flakes, which can be used in place of oatmeal in cereal, cookies and as a binding in meat loaf and other meats.

http://www.kinnikinnick.com

Miss Roben's offers excellent bread, cake, muffin, pie crust and other mixes. Miss Roben's worked with ANDI to develop ANDI Wunderbread—a terrier soft, white sandwich bread. ANDI News subscribers receive a 10% discount on their first order. They have greatly expanded their offerings. Our favorite mail-order resources!

http://www.missroben.com

Nu-World Amaranth has many amaranth products, another GF grain.

www.nuworldamaranth.com

Omega Nutrition sells everything from vitamins to nut flours. They sell some hard to find items, such as hazelnut flour and pumpkin seed spread, and are a source for natural, unprocessed coconut oil products. Omega's catalogue is also full of useful information about foods and nutrition.

www.omegaflo.com

Very Special Foods carries very unusual food items; if you are seeking foods that your child has never eaten for a strict elimination diet, this is the place to start.

http://www.specialfoods.com

Tinkyada rice pastas are available at many health food stores, but if you can't find them try their web site. Some people think their rice pastas are the best.

http://www.tinkyada.com

Dairy Substitutes

Note: Most of the "milk" products listed here are fortified with calcium and vitamin D, but you may want to supplement these as well. Some have additional nutrients added. The products below are gf/cf unless noted, but ingredients are subject to change, and there are many other suitable milk substitutes not listed, so read labels carefully and call the manufacturer when in doubt!

Vance's DariFree™:

This potato-based drink tastes good and looks like milk. It has no cholesterol, lactose, soy, rice, corn, oils or MSG. It is also excellent for baking and cooking (and is my personal favorite). Some health food stores carry DariFree™, but most people will need to order. Get it from Miss Roben's or the Gluten-Free Pantry, or order directly: 800-497-4834.

Better Than Milk®:

This tofu beverage is both gluten and casein-free. It tastes quite good, and can be used in bread and other recipes that call for "dry milk." Made by Sovex Foods (800-227-2320), it can typically be found in health food stores. Note: This product comes in two forms. Do not buy European style, it contains casein. The canisters are clearly marked.

EdenBlend:

This drink is easily found in grocery and health food stores, and comes in 32 oz. cartons. It contains water, brown rice, soybeans, kombu (seaweed), Carageenan, sea salt and calcium carbonate. Some people think it is less "beany" than straight soy milk. It looks less appealing than other "milks" as it is brownish in color. Another variety sold by Eden Foods is called EdenRice. They are similar, but EdenRice is sweetened with rice syrup that uses barley enzymes in processing. EdenBlend is a safer choice.

Pacific Ultra:

This soy beverage has no gluten hidden in the rice syrup. It contains lactobacillus acidophilus and L. bifidus.

Pacific RiceMilk

also contains lactobacillus acidophilus and L. bifidus. This rice drink is also casein and gluten-free.

Rice Dream: NOT GLUTEN-FREE!

Silk Milk

by White Wave is an excellent soy drink: thick and tasty. It comes in quart and half gallon containers and can be found in the refrigerator section of most markets or health food stores. It comes in three varieties, but only the ORGANIC (red carton) is gluten-free. Both the plain and chocolate versions are excellent.

So Nice Soyganic

Soy Milk by Soyco is similar to Silk Milk, is calcium enriched, and is gluten and dairy-free.

SoyGood:

BestLife makes a soy-based beverage called SoyGood. It is casein and gluten-free, and calcium enriched. It tastes quite a bit like milk, and can be ordered by mail order. 800-407-7238

Westsoy Plus:

This drink is very good, and although the color is a little on the yellow side, it looks appetizing. It is thick and very tasty; the fat-free version is thinner. If soy is tolerated, this is one of the better tasting drinks.

Cookbooks*

1. *The Candida Control Cookbook*, by Gail Burton (1993). Published by Aslan Publishing.

2. *The Complete Allergy Self-Help Cookbook*, by Marjorie Hurt Jones, R.N. (1984). Rodale Press.

3. *The Complete Food Allergy Cookbook, The Foods You've Always Loved Without the Ingredients You Can't Have* by Marilyn Gioannini (1995). Published by Prima Pub

4. *Dietary Intervention as a Therapy in the Treatment ofAutism and Related Developmental Disorders* by Beth and Andy Crowell (1995).

5. *Easy Bread Making for Special Diets*, by Nicolette Dumke (1995). Adapt Books: Louisville.

6. *The Gluten-Free Baker Newsletters* by Sandra Leonard, 361 Cherywood Dr., Fairborn, OH 45324-4012, e-mail: thebaker@CRIS.com

7. *The Gluten-free Gourmet* by Betty Hagman, (1991) Published by Henry Holt (Paper).

8. *More from the Gluten-free Gourmet: Delicious Dining Without Wheat* by Bette Hagman, (1994). Published by Henry Holt (Paper)

9. *The Gluten-free Gourmet Cooks Fast and Healthy: Wheat-free and Gluten-free With No Fuss and Less Fat*, by Bette Hagman, (1996). Published by Henry Holt (Paper).

10. *The Gluten-free Gourmet Bakes Bread* by Bette Hagman, (1999). Henry Holt (hardcover).

11. *Going Against the Grain*, by Phyllis Potts, (1992). Published by Central Point Publishing.

12. *Special Diet Solutions* by Carol Fenster. Savory Palate, Littleton, CO.

13. *The Wheat-free Kitchen: A Celebration of Good Foods* by Jacqueline Mallorca, Farthing Press, PO Box 471171, San Francisco, CA 94147.

ENDNOTES

1 Once we finally understood this, we took to telling uncomfortable doctors and educators that it was OK to use the 'A' word!

2 I had already removed dairy products a year before, without much effect.

3 There are many Internet lists such as this one. To subscribe, send email to: listserv@mailstrom.stjohns.edu with "subscribe autism" in the body of the mail. You can also access the postings through any Internet browser that has a "newsreader." The list name is "bit.listserv.autism" should you read the postings this way.

CHAPTER 1

1 At this time, I had no idea that Sam had any problems other than asthma, and he certainly was not on any special diet or intervention. Since that time, I have heard from many parents who report a significant improvement in language and other developmental problems during and immediately after intravenous feeding. Sam was amazingly alert and verbal right after four days of no solid food. The reintroduction of foods which we later realized were a problem for him, caused a fairly rapid descent into extremely odd behavior. At the time, we had no idea of the significance of these events.

2 Serge knew (or at least acknowledged) that there were problems long before I would or could.

3 Reports of impaired hearing are often the first clinical manifestations of autism. While audiologists generally

recognize this, they often fail to advise parents appropriately, feeling that it is only their place to confirm or rule out hearing impairment.

4 It is tragic that many sources on autism continue to describe these children as aloof, or without affect. In reality, many autistic children show a great deal of emotion. While this can and often does take the negative form of violent temper tantrums, many autistic children are very affectionate with great attachment to loved ones. Descriptions which deny this variability on the autistic spectrum do a great disservice to families, by keeping parents in denial and children from much needed intervention.

5 This refers to the *Diagnostic and Statistical Manual*, 3rd edition, revised, which was in use at the time Sam was diagnosed. It is an 800+ page book, published by the American Psychiatric Association, which serves as the bible for diagnosing mental illness. Since most mental illnesses have no medical test, the DSM lists sets of symptoms for various mental disorders. Doctors review a patient's history and behavior and compare it to accepted diagnostic guidelines. Currently, doctors are using the DSM-IV. Many autism professionals had hoped that the ubiquitous category "PDD-NOS" would be excluded from this edition of the manual, but it was actually expanded somewhat.

6 Doris Rapp has specialized in treating children with food and environmental allergies, and is the author of several books, including *Is This Your Child?* On the talk show promoting her book, Dr. Rapp showed videotapes of children who had been given an extract of a food that they were allergic to. These children became wild, aggressive, uncontrollable. Their behavior looked so much like Sam's when he was raging, that I felt dietary experimentation was worth a try.

7 A "rough day" was the teacher's euphemism for "awful." She knew it was too harsh to actually say, and I always felt grateful at her use of *rough* instead. Everyone who spent time with Sam, including his bus driver, took up this phrase as well.

8 Sam's teacher experimented with a slim-chair to teach Sam that he could practice this odd behavior, but only if he had earned a break, and only in a particular place. This place was later moved to a more private spot, and eventually the rule was that he had to use the restroom or some other private place. This intervention later became the basis of his teacher's master's thesis!

CHAPTER 2

1 Like others, I believe there is truth in the saying: "Not being able to speak does not mean you have nothing to say." But there is no denying that, at least as we are able to measure it, many autistics test in the mild to profound range of mental retardation.

2 A recent Internet search turned up over 50 hospital based Ketogenic Diet programs in 33 states.

3 In 1974, the number of food additives approved for use was 2,764.

4 Neurotransmitters are chemicals that mediate the transmission of electrical signals between neurons (nerve cells) in the brain and nervous system. Some common neurotransmitters include dopamine, serotonin, catecholemine and adrenaline.

5 Another peak has been identified by yet another group of researchers, working for a large commercial firm based in the U.S. The significance of this peak for identification or treatment of some types of autism has yet to be announced while

scientists await confirmation of patents. Certainly this discovery bodes well for autism research, and possibly treatment. I hoped that more would be revealed in the coming year.

6 One might then ask why all celiacs are not also autistic. It may be that many more celiacs would have suffered neurological damage, had the typical failure to thrive not prompted early diagnosis and removal of offending proteins from the diet. But the opioid excess theory also requires a metabolic error of some sort, which causes the improper metabolism of the proteins. If true, it may be that most celiac patients do not have this additional deficiency.

7 According to Dr. Sidney Baker, autistic children very often show deficiencies in the sulfur bearing amino acids.

CHAPTER 3

1 Material cited here was found on the American Academy of Allergy and Immunology website.

2 This horrifying statistic was cited by Dr. Allan Magaziner during a talk in Lawrenceville, NJ (1997.)

3 These unusual ingredients include white sweet potato, true yams, malaria, cassava, lotus roots, artichokes, sorghum, unusual fruits and water chestnuts.

4 The Slimak children are now, several years later, able to eat whatever they want. Their diets are completely unrestricted.

5 My son tested negative for all food allergies, when given a scratch test by a pediatric allergist. We thought that many foods provoked a reaction, but Sam tested positive only for pollens and molds. Wheat and milk produced no reaction whatsoever. Because this doctor did not believe in food intolerance, for a time we were persuaded to forget about dietary interventions.

6 It is often difficult to distinguish which foods cause a reaction, either because an innocuous food is always being eaten together with a problematic one, or because some reactions are delayed.

7 For my son, removing wheat caused a nearly immediate correction of pronouns, which had been consistently confused for three years.

8 Obviously, most children on this diet will not be consuming milk. If members of your family do consume cow's milk, be sure to find out if your state requires labeling of milk which comes from cattle treated with hormones.

CHAPTER 4

1 The ARI serves several vital functions, including keeping parents informed of the latest developments (medical, educational and political). Perhaps more important, it serves as a valuable starting point for parents of newly diagnosed children to gain information about autism and alternative treatments.

2 Since that time, another parent who attended the first DAN! meeting has, along with her husband, started a funding organization devoted to raising money to fund autism research. CAN (Cure Autism Now) began funding within a year of its organization. To find out how you can help, call 1-213-549-0500, or send email to: CAN@primenet.com.

3 I was one of four parents invited to join this first meeting. Subsequent meetings have included hundreds of interested parents and physicians.

4 Write to the ARI at 4182 Adams Avenue, San Diego, CA 92166 to order the protocol, subscribe to the newsletter or make a much-needed contribution.

5 Paul Whitely, one of Shattock's colleagues, has recently begun a formal study to monitor the progress of subjects who begin a GF/CF diet after being tested in their laboratory.

6 This statistic was gleaned from a post Dr. Horvath made to an electronic bulletin board used by celiac professionals.

7 If CD is not ruled out it can only be confirmed via intestinal biopsy. If a gluten-free diet has already been implemented, these tests will not be valid, so it makes sense to run the tests prior to beginning a dietary intervention.

8 The sugars are combined into a drink; consumption of the drink is followed by a fast of several hours, and then a urine sample is collected. Since the test requires no needles, it shouldn't be too hard to get cooperation from your child. The test is performed by the Great Smokies Diagnostic Laboratory; a doctor must order the test, and will provide you with a kit of collection instructions and the necessary drink.

9 Casein, on the other hand, appears to be out of the system soon after it is no longer being eaten.

10 My son was three when I removed dairy from his diet, and five when I removed wheat. While wheat is certainly the source of most gluten in our diets, he was in effect weaned from gluten gradually. His gluten was greatly reduced but not eliminated totally until a few months later, when I also removed oats, barley and rye. Had I known that it was gluten that should be avoided, I would no doubt have taken the cold turkey approach and he probably would have shown a negative reaction of some sort. Instead, he showed immediate improvement when removed from wheat, and then continued to improve without negative reaction when the other grains were removed.

CHAPTER 5

1 Throughout these recipes I refer to milk or dry milk powder or milk substitute. The dairy lobby in this country is very strong, and the companies who make these products are not allowed to use these words in their advertising. They are generally referred to as "Non-dairy beverages," but for the purposes of drinking a white liquid that is fortified with vitamins and calcium, or cooking with a powder version of the same product I will use the word *milk*.

2 Please note that whenever a brand name is mentioned, that brand was acceptable at the time of publication. Companies change their ingredients, or the sources of their ingredients, all the time. Always read labels carefully, and if you have any doubt or question about the acceptability of the product CALL the company. All food companies are happy to answer questions about their ingredients. If you cannot be sure that a food is acceptable—don't use it!

3 Lard is another source of fat that has no dairy, corn or soy. It is generally not acceptable, however, because it contains the preservatives BHA and BHT. These should be avoided whenever possible.

4 Many parents have told me that after months (or even years) of unsuccessful toilet training, their children were trained 'overnight' within a few weeks of going GF/CF. It seems likely the problem was really one of sensory input. Once the offending proteins or foods were removed, the children first began to feel the sensation of needing to use the bathroom. The lesson had not been lost, but it had been impossible for the children to know when it should be applied. Once that impediment was removed, the old training was, for the first time, useful.